Praises for This Book and The Bragg Healthy Lifestyle

These are just a few of the thousands of testimonials we receive yearly, praising The Bragg Health Books for the rejuvenation benefits they reap – physically, mentally and spiritually. We look forward to hearing from you also.

Thanks to Paul Bragg and Bragg Books, my years of asthma were cured in only one month with The Bragg Breathing and The Healthy Lifestyle Living! – Paul Wenner, Gardenburger Creator
www.gardenburger.com

Bragg Super Power Breathing helps make the weak strong and athletes champions. – Bob Anderson, world famous coach
www.stretching.com

The Bragg Healthy Lifestyle, the vinegar drink & fasting has changed my life! I lost weight and my energy levels went through the roof. I look forward to my fasting days. I think better and am a better husband and father. Thank you Patricia and Dad, this has been a great blessing in my life. Also, we enjoyed your important health sharing at our "AOL" Conference.
– Byron H. Elton, VP Entertainment, Time Warner AOL

Thank you Patricia for our first meeting in London in 1968. You gave me your Fasting Book, it got me exercising, brisk walking and eating more wisely. You were a blessing God-sent.
– Rev. Billy Graham www.billygraham.org

When I was a young gymnastics coach at Stanford University, Paul Bragg's words and example inspired me to live a healthy lifestyle. I was twenty-three then; now I'm sixty, and my health and fitness serves as a living testimonial to Bragg's health wisdom, carried on by his dedicated health crusading daughter, Dr. Patricia Bragg. Thank you!
– Dan Millman, Author "The Way of the Peaceful Warrior"
www.danmillman.com

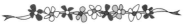

Just by paying attention to breathing, you can access new levels of health and relaxation that will benefit every area of your life.
– Deepak Chopra, M.D. www.chopra.com

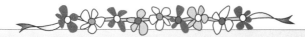

Praises for The Bragg Healthy Lifestyle

Paul Bragg saved my life at age 15 when I attended the Bragg Health Crusade in Oakland. I thank the Bragg Healthy Lifestyle for my long, healthy, active life spreading health and fitness.
– Jack LaLanne, Thankful Bragg follower for 75 years

Thanks to the ageless Bragg Health Books, they were our introduction to healthy living. We are very grateful to you and your father. – Marilyn Diamond, Co-Author "Fit For Life"

The Bragg Healthy Lifestyle and brisk walking (3X daily) for 20 minutes after meals, helped eliminate my diabetes! My whole body, blood circulation, feet and eyes have all improved. Thank you, may God continue to bless your Crusade. – John Risk, Santee, CA

As a youth I had a learning disability and was told I would never read, write or communicate normally. At 14 I dropped out of school and at 17 ended up in Hawaii surfing. My road to recovery led me to Dr. Paul Bragg who changed my life by giving me one simple affirmation to repeat: "I am a genius and I apply my wisdom." Dr. Bragg inspired me to go back to school and get my education and from there miracles happened. I've authored 54 training programs and 14 books and love to crusade around the world thanks to Bragg.
–Dr. John Demartini, Author and Dynamic Crusader (www.drdemartini.com)

For 30 years I've followed The Bragg Healthy Lifestyle - It teaches you how to take control of your health and build a healthy future.
– Mark Victor Hansen, Co-Author, "Chicken Soup for the Soul Series"

I met Paul C. Bragg on April 6, 1964 at the famous "L" Street Beach in Boston. We became instant friends. The following day he introduced me to his daughter Patricia. We have been friends ever since. Both Paul and Patricia have always been health inspirations to millions around the world, but especially to me! I gave my first public lecture with Paul and Patricia in April of '64, I was 22 then, I am now 63. Paul was always dynamic, energetic and a life-changer! Patricia has continued the Bragg Health Crusade and has more energy than any 3 people I know put together.
– Dr. David Carmos, Co-Author with Dr. Shawn Miller
"You're Never Too Old To Become Young" – www.perfecthealthnow.com

In Medical School I read Dr. Bragg's Health Books and they changed my thinking and the path of my life. I founded the Omega Institute.
– Stephan Rechtschaffen, M.D. www.eomega.org

Improper breathing is a common cause of ill health. Changing your breathing patterns can affect and improve you mentally, emotionally and physically.
– Andrew Weil, M.D. www.drweil.com

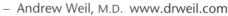

Praises for This Book and The Bragg Healthy Lifestyle

Bragg Books were my conversion to the healthy way.
– James F. Balch, M.D.,"Prescription for Nutritional Healing"

How I beat cancer, obesity, diabetes, strep and three herniated disks and excruciating pain? The answer was changing to the Bragg's Healthy Lifestyle and also doing the Super Breathing Exercises. It changed and saved my life! I had full recovery and also lost 70 lbs. I received a new life and that is just the beginning because my manhood returned that was lost to diabetes – now that's exciting! On my trip to Honolulu, Hawaii I visited the famous free Bragg Exercise Class at Waikiki Beach. I became so regenerated with a wonderful new viewpoint towards living my healthy lifestyle that I now live in Hawaii. I'm invigorated with new energy for life and living! My new purpose for living is to help others reclaim their health rights! I also want the world to join The Bragg Health Crusade. I am deeply thankful Paul and Patricia for my new healthy life!
– Len Schneider, Honolulu, Hawaii

Thank you Paul and Patricia Bragg for my simple, easy to follow Health Program. You make my day!
– Clint Eastwood, Bragg follower for over 50 years

See more Praises – page 172

We get letters daily at our Santa Barbara headquarters. We would love to receive a testimonial letter from you on any blessings, healings and changes you experienced after following The Bragg Healthy Lifestyle and this book. It's all within your grasp to be in top health. By following this book, you can reap more Super Health and a happy, longer vital life! It's never too late to begin. Studies show amazing results that were obtained with people in their 80's and 90's – Pages 6 & 34. Receive miracles with healthy nutrition, fasting and exercise! Start now!

Daily our prayers & love go out to you, your heart, mind & soul.
with love,

3 John 2   *Patricia Bragg*   Genesis 6:3

Miracles can happen every day through guidance and prayer! – Patricia Bragg

C

BRAGG HEALTH CRUSADES for 21st Century
Teaching People Worldwide to Live Healthy,
Happy, Stronger, Longer Lives for a Better World

We love sharing, teaching and giving world-wide, and you can share this love by being a partner sharing The Bragg Health Crusades and Bragg Healthy Lifestyle messages. We are dedicated with a passion to help others! We feel blessed when you and your family's lives improve through following our teachings from the Bragg Health Books and The Bragg Crusades. It makes our years of faithful service so worthwhile! We will keep sharing, and please do write us how our health teachings have helped you.

The Miracle of Fasting book has been the #1 Health book for over 18 years in Russia, the Ukraine and now Bulgaria! Why? Because we show them how to live a healthy, wholesome life for less money, and it's so easy to understand and follow. Most healthful lifestyle habits are free (good posture, clean thoughts, plain natural food, exercise and deep breathing, all of which promotes energy and health into the body). We continue to reach the multitudes worldwide with our health books and teachings, lectures, health crusades, radio and TV outreaches.

My joy and priorities come from God, Mother Nature and healthy living. I love being a health crusader and spreading health worldwide, for now it's needed more than ever! My father and I also pioneered Health TV with our program "Health and Happiness" from Hollywood. Yes – it's thrilling to be a Health Crusader and you will enjoy it also. See back pages to list names (yourself, family and friends) who you feel would benefit from receiving our free Health Bulletins!

By reading Bragg Self-Health Books you gain a new confidence that you can help yourself, family and friends to The Bragg Healthy Principles of Living! Please call your local book stores and health stores and ask for the Bragg Health Books. Prayerfully, we hope to have all stores stock the books. We do keep prices low as possible so they will be affordable and available for everyone to learn to live and enjoy a fuller, healthier, happier and longer life!

With Blessings of Health, Peace and Love,

Patricia Bragg

BRAGG HEALTH CRUSADES, America's Health Pioneers

Keep Bragg Health Crusades "Crusading" with your tax deductible donations.

Box 7, Santa Barbara, CA 93102 USA (805) 968-1020
Spreading health worldwide since 1912

BRAGG
SUPER POWER
BREATHING
for Super Health & High Energy

PAUL C. BRAGG, N.D., Ph.D.
LIFE EXTENSION SPECIALIST

and

PATRICIA BRAGG, N.D., Ph.D.
HEALTH & FITNESS EXPERT

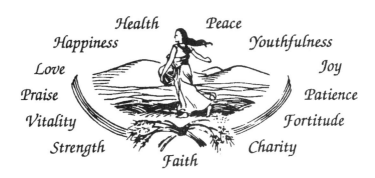

Health   *Peace*
Happiness   *Youthfulness*
Love   *Joy*
Praise   *Patience*
Vitality   *Fortitude*
Strength   *Charity*
Faith

JOIN
Bragg Health Crusades for a 100% Healthy World for All!

HEALTH SCIENCE
Box 7, Santa Barbara, California 93102 USA

World Wide Web: www.bragg.com

BRAGG
SUPER POWER
BREATHING

PAUL C. BRAGG, N.D., Ph.D.
LIFE EXTENSION SPECIALIST
and
PATRICIA BRAGG, N.D., Ph.D.
HEALTH & FITNESS EXPERT

Health Science, Box 7, Santa Barbara, California 93102
Telephone (805) 968-1020, FAX (805) 968-1001
e-mail address: books@bragg.com

Quantity Purchases: Companies, Professional Groups, Churches, Clubs, Fundraisers etc. Please contact our Special Sales Department.

To see Bragg Books, some chapters, etc. and Products on-line, visit our website at: www.bragg.com

♻ This book is printed on recycled, acid-free paper.

- REVISED AND EXPANDED -

Twenty-second printing MMV
ISBN: 0-87790-021-3

Published in the United States
HEALTH SCIENCE, Box 7, Santa Barbara, California 93102 USA

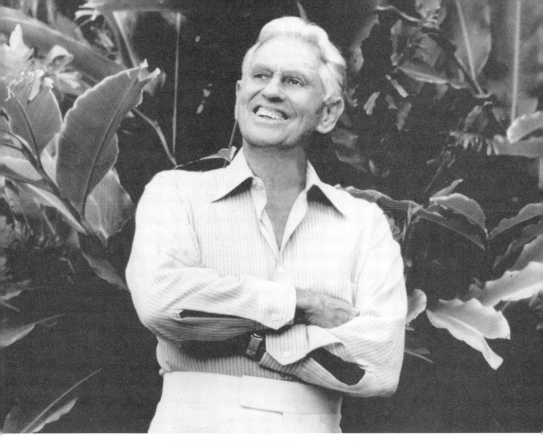

PAUL C. BRAGG, N.D., Ph.D.
World's Leading Healthy Lifestyle Authority

Paul C. Bragg's daughter Patricia and their wonderful, healthy members of the Bragg *Longer Life, Health and Happiness Club* exercise daily on the beautiful Fort DeRussy lawn, at famous Waikiki Beach in Honolulu, Hawaii. View club exercising www.bragg.com. Membership is free and open to everyone to attend any morning – Monday through Saturday, from 9 to 10:30 am – for Bragg Super Power Breathing and Health and Fitness Exercises. On Saturday there are often health lectures on how to live a long, healthy life! The group averages 75 to 125 per day, depending on the season. From December to March it can go up to 150. Its dedicated leaders have been carrying on the class for over 30 years. Thousands have visited the club from around the world and carried the Bragg Health and Fitness Crusade to friends and relatives back home. When you visit Honolulu, Hawaii, Patricia invites you and your friends to join her and the club for wholesome, healthy fellowship. She also recommends visiting the outer Islands (Kauai, Hawaii, Maui, Molokai) for a fulfilling, healthy vacation.

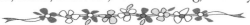

To maintain good health, normal weight and increase the good life of radiant health, joy and happiness, the body must be exercised properly (stretching, walking, aerobics, jogging, running, biking, swimming, deep breathing, good posture, etc.) and nourished wisely with healthy foods. – Paul C. Bragg

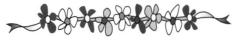

Our Favorite Quotes We Share with You . . .
where space allows. We all need inspiring, informative words of wisdom to help guide us in our daily living.

Breathing is the movement of spirit and energy within the body; and working with breathing is a form of spiritual practice. – Andrew Weil, M.D.

Man is composed of such elements as vital breath, deeds, thoughts and the senses. – The Upanishads

Here's a wise ancient Turkish saying: No matter how far you've gone down on a wrong road, turn back and get on the right road!

Dream big, think big, but enjoy the small miracles of everyday life.

When you live A Healthy Lifestyle *you can help activate your own powerful internal defense arsenal and maintain it at top efficiency. However, bad or sloppy breathing habits make it harder for your body to fight off illness.*

Every year I live I am more convinced that the waste of life lies in the love we have not given, the powers we have not used. – Mary Cholomondeley

When health is absent, wisdom cannot reveal itself, art cannot become manifest, strength cannot be exerted. Wealth is useless, and reason is powerless. – Herophiles, 300 B.C.

If you truly love Nature, you will find Beauty everywhere. – Vincent Van Gogh

God will not change the condition of men, until they change what is in themselves. – Koran

I cannot overstate the importance of the habit of quiet meditation and prayer for more health of body, mind and spirit. – Patricia Bragg

The natural healing force within us is the greatest force in getting well. – Hippocrates, Father of Medicine

When you live The Bragg Healthy Lifestyle you can help activate your own powerful internal health defense arsenal and continually maintain it at top efficiency. However, if you continue unhealthy eating and living habits, it is harder for your body to fight off illness! – Paul C. Bragg

Becoming aware of your breathing makes you more open to life's experiences. It gives you the resilience to cope with life's challenges and to enjoy its pleasures. You will learn to overcome the weariness that follows periods of poor breathing, to restore the loss of energy, and start experiencing full vitality as an unavoidable consequence of fuller breathing. – Carola Speads

ii

Super Power Breathing

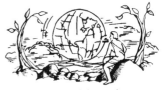

*To preserve health is a moral and religious duty, for health is the
basis for all social virtues. We can't be as useful when not well.*
– Dr. Samuel Johnson, Father of Dictionaries.

Contents

Chapter 1: Super Power Breathing for Super Energy 1

Do You Know How to Breathe? 1
Super Power Breathing is High Vibration Living 1
High Vibration Energy Produces Achievers 2
Super Power Breathing Increases Energy 2
It's Never Too Late to Improve 3
Most Live at Medium Vibration Rate 3
The Miracle Surge of the Second Wind 4
Shallow Breathing Causes Premature Ageing 4
Premature Ageing (Graphic) 5
Paul & Patricia Lift Weights (Photo) 6
Super Deep Breathing For Super Power Living 6

Chapter 2: Oxygen and Your Health 7

Oxygen Starvation 7
Life-Giving Oxygen – Invisible Staff of Life 8
The Heart and Blood Vessel Circulatory System (Graphic) 8
Oxygen Powers the Human Machine 9
Oxygen is Carried by the Bloodstream 9
Blood – Your Miracle River of Life 10
Super Power Breathing Detoxifies and Purifies Your Blood 11
Shallow Breathers Self-Poison Themselves 12

Chapter 3: The Way You Breathe Affects your Life 13

When you Breathe Deeply and Fully You Live Longer and more Healthy 13
Super Deep Breathing Improves the Brain 14
Give Thanks to Your Miracle-Working Lungs 14
The Lower Respiratory System (Graphic) 15
Path of Breath (Graphic) 15
Mechanics of Breathing (Graphic) 15
The Lungs Are Nature's Miracle Breathers 16
You have Lungs – Fill Them Up 17
The Importance of Clean Air to Health 17
Live Longer Breathing *Clean Air Deeply* 18

*The best service a book can render you is, to impart truth,
but to make you think it out for yourself.* – Elbert Hubbard

Remember: "It is NEVER too late to be what you might have been!"

Contents

Chapter 4: Smoking – A Deadly Habit 19

Stop Smoking – Save Your Lungs and Life 20
Smoking is Robbing Millions of their Sight 20
Teens Talk About Stopping Smoking 21
Quit Smoking – See the Difference it Makes! (List) 22
Fast Return to Health When You Stop Smoking (Chart) 22
Deadly Smoking Facts! (List) 23
What Deadly Smoking Does to You and Those Around You 24

Chapter 5: The Common Cold – The Body's Miracle Cleanser 25

Colds Clean Out Mucus and Toxins 25
The Body Self-Cleanses, Repairs and Heals 26
Colds and Oxygen are Great Cleansers 26
Oxygen Cleanses and Nourishes 27

Chapter 6: Your Miracle Nose – Pathway to the Lungs 29

We Mostly Breathe Through the Nose 29
Your Nose is a Natural Air-Filtration System 30
Sinusitis Causes Breathing and Infection Problems 30
Blocked Sinuses Breed Health Problems 31
Herbs Bring Relief and Promote Healing 31
Solve Sinus and Allergy Problems 32
Most Common Food Allergies (List) 32
Nosebleeds 33
Self-test For Specific Problem Foods 33
Mind Food For Thought 34

Chapter 7: Unhealthy Homes & Buildings 35

Toxic Building Materials 35
Formaldehyde Gives Off Toxic Vapors 36
Beware of Invisible Radon Dangers 36
Healthy Home Environment is Important 37
Having a Healthy, Safe Home and More 38
Asthma From Our Environments 38
Treating Asthma Naturally 39
Self-Health Care For the Lungs 40

Chapter 8: Your Diaphragm is the Key to Breathing 41

Bragg Super Power Breathing 41
Diaphragmatic Versus Chest Breathing 42
Internal Massage by Diaphragmatic Action 43
Bragg Super Power Breathing Calms the Nervous System 44
The Ayurvedic Health and Fitness Lifestyle 44
Ancient Yoga Breathing Promotes Health 45
Bad Nutrition – #1 Cause of Sickness 45
The Posture Chart (Graphic) 46

Learning is finding out what you knew already. Doing is demonstrating that you know it. Teaching is reminding others that they know it just as well as you! You are all learners, doers and teachers. – Richard Bach

Contents

Chapter 9: The Importance of Doctor Good Posture 47

Sit, Stand and Walk Tall for Good Health! (Graphic) 47
Posture Can Make of Break Your Health! 48
Your Health Friend is Doctor Posture 48
Backaches Afflict 31 Million Americans 49
Learn to Stand, Sit and Walk Tall For Body Strength and Super Health .. 50
Don't Cross Your Legs – It's Unhealthy 51
Which Posture Do You Have? 52
Wear Loose, Comfortable Clothing 52
Bragg Posture Exercise Brings Miracles 52
Cold Water Swimmers and Fit and Ageless 53
Opera Singers, Ballet Dancers and Athletes are Deep Breathers 54
Diaphragmatic Breathing: Secret of Dancing Greats 54
Normalize Your Figure With Good Posture & Exercise 55
Good Posture – First Step to Healthy Living 56
No One Can Breathe for You 57

Chapter 10: Preparing for Bragg Super Power Breathing ... 57

Overcoming the Effects of Bad Breathing 57
Practice Bragg Posture Exercises Every Day 58
Stomach Muscles Need These Exercises 59
Diaphragm Exercise 60
Singing – Breathing Exercise 61
Candle – Breathing Exercise 61
Arm Pumping – Breathing Exercise 61
Wise Thoughts for Wise Healthy Living 62

Chapter 11: What is Bragg Super Power Breathing? 63

Basic Scientific Natural Laws 63
Bragg Breathing Stimulates Pituitary Gland 64
Fresh Air and Warmth are Necessary 65
Air Baths Are Health Builders 66
Breathe Through the Mouth and Nose 66

Chapter 12: Bragg Super Power Breathing Exercises 67

Exercise #1 – The Cleansing Breath 67
Exercise #2 – The Super Power Brain Breath 68
Exercise #3 – The Super-Kidney Breath 69
Exercise #4 – Regulations the Bowels 69
Exercise #5 – Filling the Lungs 70
Exercise #6 – The Super Power Liver Cleansing Breath 70
Exercise #7 – Heart Strengthener 71
Faithfulness Counts Towards Super Health 72

*The breathing rhythm has three components: exhalation – pause –
inhalation. The pause fulfills a double purpose: a resting from the effort of
the inhalation and a rallying of the energy needed for the next inhalation.
The pause, therefore, is not an idle period when nothing is happening,
the pause is a vital phase in the breathing process. – Carola Speads*

v

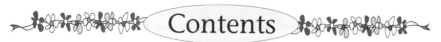

Contents

Chapter 13: Learning Breath Control **73**

You Enjoy More Health and Happiness 73

Evening and Bedtime Routines 73

Deep, Full Breathing Helps Relieve Pain 73

Heed Warning Pains – Eliminate Cause 74

Exercise Relieves Varicose Veins & Leg Swelling 75

Power Breathing & Brisk Walking Exercise 75

Brisk Walking is the King of Exercise 76

Walking Posture (Graphic) 76

Miracle - Walking Builds New Blood Vessels........................ 76

Super Power Breathing Makes Exercise Fun 77

Super Power Breathing Calms the Nerves 77

B-Complex & Magnesium Improves Breathing & Soothes Nerves 78

Deep Breathing Helps Respiratory Ailments 78

America's National "Sleep Debt" 79

Getting Enough Sleep Lately? 80

Healthful Tips for Sound, Recharging Sleep 80

Relief for the Stuffy Noses & the Snorer in the House 81

Help for Bronchitis and Asthma 81

Help for Asthma Attacks 82

Reduce Asthma Trouble Triggers 82

Controlled Deep Full Breathing Exercise 83

Diaphragmatic Panting Breathing Exercise 83

Practicing Exercises During Pregnancy 84

Benefits Mother and Baby During Pregnancy 84

One-Breath Meditation Works Miracles............................. 84

Chapter 14: Breathing Exercises to Enjoy for More Energy . **85**

Posture Breathing Exercise 85

Super Power Breathing for Fresh, New Air 86

Rejuvenation Breathing Exercise 86

Exercise to Increase Lung's Air Space 87

Exercise for Flexible, Youthful Rib Cage 87

Exercise to Maximize Chest Area 88

Breathing Exercise for Lower Lungs 88

Deep Breathing Promotes Better Sleep 89

Stop Procrastinating – Start Exercising Daily 89

Start the 10-Minute Trick – It Works Miracles 90

Chapter 15: Oxygen Depletion and Air Pollution **91**

The Urgent Problems of Air Pollution 91

What Is Smog? 91

Smog is a Deadly Health Hazard 92

Dangerous Ground -level Ozone Smog 93

Clean Air Act Benefits and Costs 93

I conceive that a knowledge of books is the basis on which all other knowledge rests.
– George Washington, First U.S. President, 1789-1797

Contents

Let's Clean Up Our Air! 94
We Need the Clean Air Act! 94
Healthful Solutions to Air Pollution 95
Clean the Air in Your Home or Office 95
Vitamin E Rich Foods (Chart) 97

Chapter 16: Doctor Natural Foods 97

Vitamin E – Nature's Health Miracle 97
Vitamin E – Your Cardiovascular's Guardian 98
Add Wonder-Working Vitamin E 99
Bragg Family's Favorite Cornmeal Recipe 99
Phytochemicals – Nature's Miracles Help Prevent Cancer (Chart) 101
Healthy Eating Gives You More Super Oxygen, Energy & Health 101
The Bragg Health Lifestyle Promotes Super Health and Super Energy! . 101
Healthy Snack Munching 102
Power Salad for Lunch = Power All Day 102
Vegetable Proteins % Chart 102

Chapter 17: Healthy Schedule of 12 Meals Per Week 105

Bragg Famous recipes 106
Enjoy Healthy, Balanced Variety for Dinner 107
Eliminating Meat is Healthiest 108
Do Not Poison Your Body with Foodless Foods and Harmful Drinks! 109
Avoid All Dangerous Embalmers – Preservatives 110
Never Use Salt It's a Slow Killer! 111
Pure Water – Essential for Health! 112
Fast 1 Day Each Week for Inner Cleansing 114
Distilled Water is the #1 Health Drink 115
Keep Fluoride and All its Toxic Risks Out of Your Water 115
Healthy Beverages and Recipes 116
Juice Fast – Introduction to Water Fast 117
Powerful Juice Combinations (List) 118
Food and Product Summary 119
Enjoy Super Health with Natural Foods 119
Benefits from The Joys of Fasting (List) 120
Avoid These Processed, Refined, Harmful Foods (List) 121
Phytochemicals – Nature's Miracle Workers 122
Enjoy Healthy Fiber for Super Health 122

Chapter 18: Powerful Benefits of Super Power Breathing . 123

A Strong Mind in a Strong Body 123
Super Oxygen Breathing for Super-Living 124
The Advantages of Super Power Breathing 124
The Bronchial Tree (Graphic) 126

*Habits can be right or wrong, good or bad, healthy or unhealthy,
rewarding or unrewarding, powerful for good, or powerful for bad. The
right or wrong habits, decisions, actions, words and deeds are up to you.
Wisely choose your habits, as they can make or break you!*

Contents

Chapter 19: Keep the Oxygen Coming 127
Heimlich Maneuver Jumpstarts the Lungs 128
Heimlich Helps Save Drowning Victims 128
Heimlich Maneuver Helps Combat Asthma 129
First Aid for Choking & Drowning Victims 130
Heimlich Maneuver Stops Asthma Attacks 131

Chapter 20: Doctor Fresh Air 133
We are Miracle Air Breathing Machines 134
Indian Holy Men Practice Deep, Slow Breathing 135
Deep Super Power Breathing 136
Healthy Walking Also Helps Solve Problems 137
Healthy Heart Habits for a Long, Vital Life (Book Excerpt) 138

Chapter 21: Doctor Rest 139
Enjoy Rest & Naps – It's Not a Crime to Relax! 140
Sleep the Miracle Recharger 141
Healthy Lifestyle Promotes Sound Sleep 141
Life is to be Savored and Enjoyed, Not Hectic 142
Love Mother Nature and Yourself Daily 143
Tips for Healthy, Peaceful Living 144

Chapter 22: Doctor Exercise 145
Exercise Promotes Healthy Elimination 146
Enjoy Brisk Walks for Healthy Long Life 146
Walking is the King of Exercise 147
The Importance of Abdominal Exercises 148
Should We Exercise During Fasting? 148
Fasting Promotes Health & Energy 149
Do These Exercises Daily 150
The Muscles of the Human Body – Front & Back View (Graphic) 151

Chapter 23: Doctor Gentle Sunshine 153
Chlorophyll is Miraculous Liquid Sunshine 154
Gentle Sunbathing Works Miracles! 154
Doctor Healing Sunshine Saved Bragg's Life 155
Boron: Miracle Trace Mineral For Healthy Bones 156

Chapter 24: Alternative Health Therapies & Massage 157-160
Chapter 25: Health Alternatives for Breathing Problems . 161
Drugs – Not Always Necessary for Recovery 161
Don't Accept Breathing Problems 161
Pollution Affects Breathing 162

Index 167

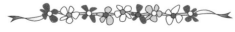

A fool thinks he needs no advice, but a wise man listens to others – Proverbs 12:15

*With improving the body's oxygenation and energy
utilization at the cellular level, you are strengthening
the immune system which is the bodyguard of your health.*

Keep Biologically Healthy & Youthful With Super Power Breathing, Exercise and Good Nutrition

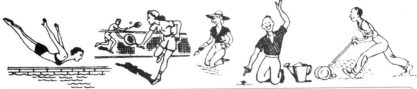

Always remember you have the following important reasons for following The Bragg Healthy Lifestyle:

- The ironclad laws of Mother Nature and God.
- Your common sense, which tells you that you are doing right.
- Your aim to make your health better and your life longer.
- Your resolve to prevent illness so that you may enjoy life.
- Make an art of healthy living; you will be youthful at any age.
- You will retain your faculties and be hale, hearty, active and useful far beyond the ordinary length of years.
- You will also possess superior mental and physical powers!

WANTED – For Robbing Health & Life

KILLER Saturated Fats	CHOKER Hydrogenated Fats
CLOGGER Salt	DEADEYED Devitalized Foods
DOPEY Caffeine	HARD WATER Inorganic Minerals
PLUGGER Frying Pan	JERKY Turbulent Emotions
DEATH-DEALER Drugs	CRAZY Alcohol
GREASY Overweight	SMOKY Tobacco
HOGGY Overeating	LOAFER Laziness

What Wise Men Say

Wisdom does not show itself so much in precept as in life – a firmness of mind and mastery of the appetite. – Seneca

I saw few die of hunger – of eating, a hundred thousand. – Ben Franklin

Govern well thy appetite, lest Sin surprise thee, and her black attendant, Death. – Milton

Your health is your wealth. – Paul C. Bragg

Our prayers should be for a sound mind in a healthy body. – Juvenal

Health is a blessing that money cannot buy. – Izaak Walton

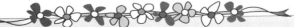

The natural healing force within us is the greatest force in getting well. – Hippocrates, Father of Medicine, 400 BC

Of all the knowledge, the one most worth having is knowledge about health! The first requisite of a good life is to be a healthy person. – Herbert Spencer

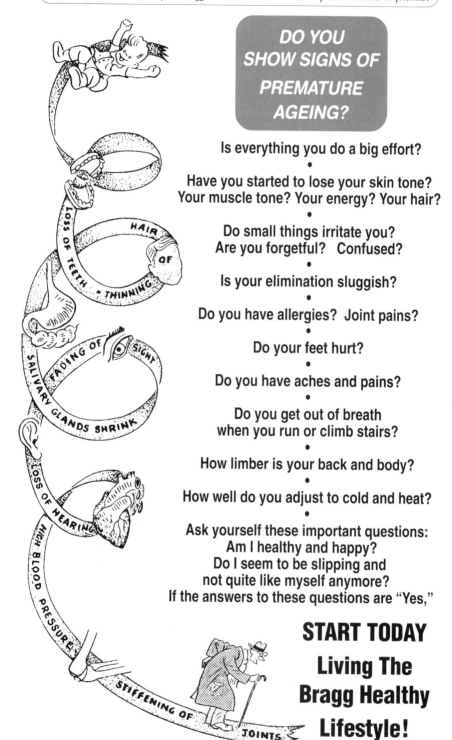

DO YOU SHOW SIGNS OF PREMATURE AGEING?

Is everything you do a big effort?

Have you started to lose your skin tone?
Your muscle tone? Your energy? Your hair?

Do small things irritate you?
Are you forgetful?   Confused?

Is your elimination sluggish?

Do you have allergies? Joint pains?

Do your feet hurt?

Do you have aches and pains?

Do you get out of breath
when you run or climb stairs?

How limber is your back and body?

How well do you adjust to cold and heat?

Ask yourself these important questions:
Am I healthy and happy?
Do I seem to be slipping and
not quite like myself anymore?
If the answers to these questions are "Yes,"

START TODAY
Living The
Bragg Healthy
Lifestyle!

X

He who understands Mother Nature walks with God.

Chapter 1

Super Power Breathing For Super Energy

Do You Know How to Breathe?

The breath of life means exactly what it says: To breathe is to live; not to breathe is to die. A human can exist without food for weeks, go without water for days, but one can't exist for more than a few minutes without air!

This fact is so obvious and breathing is so automatic that most people take it for granted. *Yet, <u>do you really know how to breathe</u>?* Stop and think about it. Do you really know how your lungs function? Do you use these marvelous organs to their fullest? The way you use your lungs controls your life, your health, your looks, your energy, your resistance to disease – your very life span!

Super Power Breathing – The Path To High Vibration Energy Living

As health specialists with over a century of combined effort, we have developed techniques for measuring mental and physical energy in humans. Everyone lives at a certain rate of vibration. The human body is capable of reaching a high vibration energy level; unfortunately very few ever master what it takes to achieve it. Why? Because only a few know how to generate, utilize and replenish their full capacity of body and mind energy.

High vibration energy people are doers and achievers. They display seemingly inexhaustible vitality and stamina, creative power and/or athletic ability of the highest quality. They never seem to tire. They perform mental and physical tasks without strain or excessive emotion. To high vibration achievers, everything seems easy and effortless because they have more vital power.

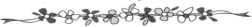

The Bragg Super Power Breathing habit of taking longer, slower, deeper breaths helps produce more energy and a more vital, youthful, longer life for you!
– Paul C. Bragg, N.D., Ph.D. Pioneer Health Crusader

High Vibration Energy Produces Achievers

This natural energy produces contented people who see the humorous side of life: full of personal magnetism and enthusiasm, high vibration energy people are a joy to be with because they have happy dispositions. They are free from depressions and mental blocks, and are well-adjusted people who enjoy more fulfilling, healthy and happy lives. What is their secret? How do they live at a superior rate of high vibration energy? The answer is simple: such people consume large amounts of oxygen. They breathe deeply and fully, utilizing every square inch of their lung capacity. Ample oxygen combined with a healthy lifestyle does bring miracles.

The more oxygen you breathe into your lungs, the more energy you will have. This creates a higher rate of vibration. It's very much like a fire in an open burning fireplace – the more oxygen the fire gets, the brighter it will burn. The less oxygen it gets, the less heat and more unwanted smoke it generates – and soon the fire dies.

Super Power Breathing Increases Energy

At age 16, my father, Paul C. Bragg, was diagnosed with a *hopeless* case of tuberculosis. Yet by age 18 he was cured and became a successful athlete. During those two years he was under the care of the great Swiss physician Dr. August Rollier. This wise doctor gave Dad a new lease on life with a regimen of all-natural healing methods. Using only pure distilled water, good nutrition, an apple cider vinegar drink, sunshine, fresh air, deep breathing and regular exercise, his body was able to cure itself with healthy natural living. After being healed, my father made a life-long pact with God to share his healthy lifestyle message with millions worldwide and he has!

Paul C. Bragg became a great-great-grandfather. He could out last most people half his age or less in any competition requiring energy and stamina. He easily typed for hours without mental or physical fatigue. He enjoyed hiking, jogging, biking, swimming, lifting weights, surfing, playing tennis and the challenge of climbing the highest mountains around the world.

It's Never Too Late to Improve

My father kept himself at a high rate of mental and physical vibration by supplying his body with the correct fuel: natural, healthy "live" foods and, above all, ample super power oxygen. He continually helped people in all walks of life – musicians, singers, writers, artists, doctors, lawyers, athletes, office workers and homemakers – to achieve a superior state of high vibration energy so they could enjoy Bragg Healthy Living. The basic source of super-oxygen-vibration is knowing how to deeply fill your lungs with oxygen. Everyone is born with this capacity, but only a few retain this deep breathing habit naturally throughout life like athletes and singers do.

Whatever your age, it's never too late to learn how to increase your energy with the Bragg System of Super Power Breathing. After faithfully following the breathing exercises in this book, you too can soon learn how to fill your lungs with energy-producing, super power oxygen. You will enjoy the thrill of this great oxygen stimulation. It's far more potent than any toxic artificial stimulants such as alcohol, coffee, tea, cola and soft drinks and drugs. Plus oxygen has no side effects! In fact, deep oxygen stimulation can add up to a longer, healthier and fuller, happier lifetime.

Most Live at Low to Medium Vibration

People who live at a low to medium rate of vibration attain limited levels of vitality, both mentally and physically. While they have a fine capacity for work and play, they aren't capable of the sustained effort achieved by those who have high vibration energy. Low to medium vibration energy people easily tire and lack endurance, particularly when under stress. Exhaustion induced by tension and strain forces this type of person to stop and rest and even give up.

People living even at a medium vibration rate simply don't get enough vital oxygen to give them that extra push to keep going under physical, mental or emotional pressures. Under extreme pressure they *run out of gas* and lack the high vibration energy that deep power breathing provides to make this additional effort.

3

The Miracle Surge of the Second Wind

Why can't they get their *second wind*? It is because they are not using the full capacity of their miracle lungs for energy-producing oxygen. That is the difference between the person who lives at the high vibration level and those who draw on only a medium rate of vibration.

At a high rate of vibration, when you consume your full quota of oxygen, you are able to get your *second wind*. You feel stronger than when you started your effort. This miracle *second wind* is what makes high achievers. Champion athletes, statesmen and women, writers, singers, actors, dancers and go-getters are equally high achievers.

When you learn to use the full capacity of your lungs through the Bragg System of Super Power Breathing, you will experience this wonderful stimulation of the *second wind*. Just when you think you have run out of energy, this sudden renewal of strength occurs. This is an experience truly difficult to describe. When you feel you cannot take another step, that your brain power is all gone, that your thinking is befuddled, then suddenly a great surge of energy courses through your entire body. You soon feel as fresh as, or even stronger than when you started! What a tremendous sensation! When you do this breathing correctly you can experience this amazing *second wind*. Many Olympic champions won their gold medals using Bob Anderson's wise help – the world's leading stretching coach (book on Amazon.com) who teaches Bragg Super Power Breathing at seminars worldwide.

Shallow Breathing Causes Premature Ageing

Regrettably, even the people who live at a medium rate of vibration are in the minority. In our modern world, most people are only half alive, existing merely at a very low rate of physical and mental vibration. Look around you – this includes people of all ages – from the early teens to the late 80s (if they live that long).

Babies use their lungs as Mother Nature intended, but soon they acquire the unnatural, *civilized* habit of shallow breathing. They begin to use only the top part of their lungs.

Gardenburger Creator Thanks Bragg Books
Cured His Asthma in a Month

Paul Wenner, the *Gardenburger* Creator, says his early years as a youth with asthma were so bad he would stand at the window praying to breathe through the night and stay alive. A miracle happened when as a young teenager he read the Bragg Books – *The Miracle of Fasting*, *Breathing* and *Healthy Lifestyle* and his years of asthma were cured in only one month. Paul became so inspired he wanted to be a health crusader like Paul Bragg & Patricia – and he has! *Gardenburgers are now sold worldwide.*
Visit web: www.gardenburger.com

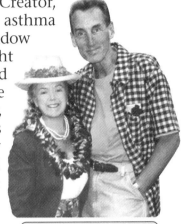
Patricia with Paul Wenner

Faith and Vision Create Miracles

Those happy, healthy, strong and vigorous people – those people who accomplish greatness – all those of faith, possess a deep spiritual philosophy. They believe that their lives are protected by a Power greater than their own. They believe there is a destiny which guides their lives. Nothing can thwart them! Following the wise Eternal Laws of God and Mother Nature you can accomplish great miracles!

Patricia's "Angel Gift" to You

Here's your own "Pocket Angel" to be with you night and day –
To guide, protect, and show you right from wrong, and help you heal your life- physically, mentally, emotionally & spiritually with Angel Love.

(Zerox page, cut out Angel Strip, fold & keep in wallet.)

> *They that wait upon the Lord shall renew their strength; They shall mount up with wings as eagles; They shall run, and not be weary; And they shall walk, and not faint.*

I cannot overstate the importance of the habit of quiet prayer and meditation for more health of body, mind, and spirit. "In quietness shall be your strength." – Isaiah 30:15

The natural healing force within you is the greatest force in getting well.
– Hippocrates, Father of Medicine, 400 B.C.

What wound did ever heal but by gentle degrees. – William Shakespeare

Paul and Patricia Bragg Lift Weights 3 Times Weekly

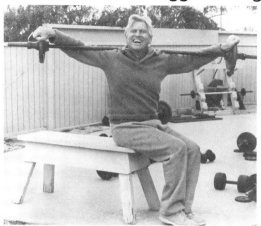

Dr. Fiatarone's Boston study and others have proven that weight-lifting rejuvenates oldsters. Try it– it works for us and others! Studies conclude: "A 3 day-a-week weight-training program is capable of inducing a dramatic increase in health and muscle strength in frail men and women even up to 96 years of age."

Visit website: www2.fhs.usd.edu.au/ess/fiatarone

Enjoy Bragg Super Power Breathing For Super-Charged Powerful Living

Shallow breathing starves the body of the oxygen it needs to be vitally alive. That's why there are so many people – from teenagers to oldsters – crowding doctors' offices, clinics, sanitariums, hospitals and convalescent homes. They drag themselves through life, seeking imaginary quick-fixes from artificial remedies in the form of laxatives, painkillers, tonics, sleeping pills and other popular, advertised over-the-counter drugs.

Oxygen-starved people are usually nervous and suffer from unnecessary worries as well as physical ills. Millions go to bed exhausted and wake up tired. They suffer from headaches, constipation, indigestion, muscular aches and pains, stiff joints, sore backs and feet, painful teeth and receding gums, poor eyesight and hearing, loss of memory, inflamed throats and respiratory ailments such as bronchitis, asthma, sinus infections and emphysema.

These health miseries and the loss of healthy bodily functions (which are often attributed to *ageing*) plague millions and can take them to an early grave. They suffer and die needlessly – simply because they don't live a healthy lifestyle and most importantly, learn to breathe deep and fully! It seems incredible, but with Super Power Breathing miracles happen! Prove it to yourself! Life and health are priceless and should be treasured.

Chapter 2

Oxygen and Your Health

Oxygen Starvation

Suppose you are very hungry and sit down to enjoy a well-planned, nourishing meal . . . but as soon as you have eaten only a few bites of the food, someone snatches it away and tells you that you can't have any more! What would you think of the food-snatcher?

This is exactly what you do to yourself when you shallow breathe as most people do, using only ¼ to ⅓ of your lung capacity! This starves your body more than if you were depriving it of food. You are robbing your body of its most vital, invisible nourishment – oxygen.

Oxygen is essential to the ionization process, in which food molecules are broken down into nutrients suitable for the body's vital needs. Without sufficient oxygen your body cannot properly utilize the food you eat and drink, no matter how basically nourishing the food may be.

With an insufficient supply of life-giving oxygen, your bloodstream becomes saturated with poisonous carbon dioxide and other toxic wastes. It transports these toxins throughout your body (collecting more en route), thereby suffocating your cells (also dulling brain cells), instead of rejuvenating them with sufficient life-giving oxygen.

Your brain, which requires three times more oxygen than the rest of your body, suffers first. Philip Rice, M.D., who is a specialist with delinquent children, warns:

> *"55% of the delinquent behavior in minors can be attributed to oxygen starvation."*

Oxygen starvation is caused by shallow breathing, sedentary habits and lack of exercise and fresh air. Educators who are alarmed about the decrease in the average student's IQ would do well to promote school physical education, exercise, sports and open windows. Tests and analyses are not brain food, but life-giving oxygen is!

7

Life-Giving Oxygen – Invisible Staff of Life

You can perform a simple demonstration by lighting two candles and placing them side by side, a few inches apart. Now partially cover one candle with a glass . . . watch how small and pale this flame becomes. If you cover the candle completely with the glass, the flame will go out in a few seconds. That is what happens in your body when you deprive it of life-giving oxygen.

THE HEART AND BLOOD VESSEL CIRCULATORY SYSTEM

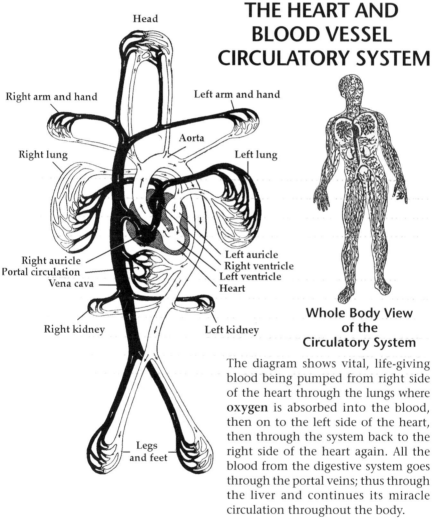

Head

Right arm and hand

Left arm and hand

Aorta

Right lung

Left lung

Right auricle
Portal circulation
Vena cava

Left auricle
Right ventricle
Left ventricle
Heart

Right kidney

Left kidney

Legs and feet

Whole Body View of the Circulatory System

The diagram shows vital, life-giving blood being pumped from right side of the heart through the lungs where **oxygen** is absorbed into the blood, then on to the left side of the heart, then through the system back to the right side of the heart again. All the blood from the digestive system goes through the portal veins; thus through the liver and continues its miracle circulation throughout the body.

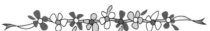

The Color Doppler flow imaging test (safe, non-evasive imaging ultrasound) shows a clear profile that checks the entire blood vessel system simultaneously. When needed, doctors check for possible blood slow-down and blockages.

Oxygen Powers the Human Machine

The human body is a marvelous and intricate mechanism for the production of mental and physical energy. Oxygen is this mechanism's power source. Your body begins to function with your first breath and continues until your last. How well it functions depends on how well you supply it with powerful oxygen.

As in any heat or combustion engine, **oxygen is essential to the production of energy in your body.** Every flame consists of the union of oxygen with other elements. The gasoline that fuels your car, the natural gas or coal in a heater or furnace and the wood in a fireplace or stove all contain latent energy. This energy cannot be released to produce heat or power until its elements are broken down and united with oxygen.

This human body process is called metabolism. The food you eat contains latent energy, but it's of absolutely no use to you without oxygen. To determine the general health of our bodies, we can test the rate of our basal metabolism. This rate is determined in a laboratory by measuring the oxygen we use while our body is resting.

As long as you live, the body mechanism operates continuously. Even while asleep, your lungs and heart, kidneys, liver and other major organs, as well as circulatory and nervous systems, must continue to function. The amount of energy you need depends, of course, upon your mental, as well as physical activities. **The release of the energy you need depends upon your intake of oxygen and your general well-being.**

Oxygen is Carried by the Bloodstream

Every one of the over 300 trillion cells in your body demands a continuous flow of life-giving oxygen in order to stay alive, do its job and remain healthy. This oxygen supply is carried in your bloodstream by the red blood cells. There are millions of these red cells in every drop of your blood (each body averages about 35 trillion).

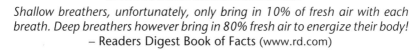

Shallow breathers, unfortunately, only bring in 10% of fresh air with each breath. Deep breathers however bring in 80% fresh air to energize their body!
– Readers Digest Book of Facts (www.rd.com)

Blood – Your Miracle River of Life!

The blood circulates in an average network of around 60,000 miles of blood vessels that reach every cell in the body, from those of the heart itself to the top of the scalp and to the tips of the fingers and toes. The average individual has about five to six quarts of blood circulating throughout their vast body network.

During rest or inactivity the blood makes one round trip per minute. During strenuous activity or exercise, however, it may make as many as eight or nine round trips per minute in order to supply the necessary fuel and oxygen for increased energy, and to help remove waste products and toxins from the body.

The blood vessels that carry blood from the heart are known as arteries. Those that return blood to the heart are veins. Both vary greatly in size and are organized just like streams, brooks and creeks flowing into a river, which joins a larger river. <u>Your body is a miracle.</u>

The smallest blood vessels are called capillaries. They are so tiny that most are visible only under a microscope! Through these capillaries the last of the food and oxygen is given off and the return trip is made via the veins, which carry the oxygen-depleted blood and toxic wastes back to the heart for purification. En route to the heart, however, most of the water-soluble wastes are transferred to the kidneys for elimination through the urine. Poisonous carbon dioxide gas, a major residue of energizing oxidation, is brought back to the heart to be expelled through the lungs.

Blood is the river of life that flows through the human body. We cannot live without it. The heart pumps blood to all our body's cells, supplying them with oxygen and food.

To reduce your risk of heart disease, boost your good blood cholesterol and reduce the bad. This can be done by following a healthy low-fat diet and reducing total cholesterol intake. Exercise also boosts good cholesterol, as does being trim and fit and, of course, not smoking. And don't expect results overnight! It takes time for exercising and diet to bring about a significant change in your cholesterol level. But be faithful and diligent – it works!
– UC Berkeley Wellness Letter (www.berkeleywellness.com)

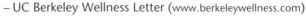

Super Power Breathing
Detoxifies and Purifies Your Blood

The carbon dioxide collected from all parts of the body gives the blood a blueish color when it is returned through the veins to the heart. There it enters the right auricle, the heart's upper chamber. After the auricle fills with blood, the valve into the right ventricle (lower chamber) opens, allowing the blood to pass into the ventricle. When the valve closes, the ventricle's strong muscles contract, sending blood to the lungs.

As blood travels through the capillary network in the lungs' air sacs, it discharges its load of carbon dioxide. It turns a healthy, bright red again as it absorbs the vital, life-giving oxygen before it immediately returns to the hearts left auricle. From there the blood flows into the left ventricle and by valve action is pumped vigorously into the body's largest artery, the aorta. Leaving the aorta, the blood then travels throughout the body via a vast arterial network – taking its life-giving oxygen and nutrients to every body cell to keep you healthy.

It is the shorter or *lesser* circulation – from the heart to the lungs and back – that is so vital to detoxifying and purifying the bloodstream. If the lungs are only partially filled with air, only part of the bloodstream can be cleansed. The blood which passes through the capillaries of empty air sacs cannot get rid of its carbon dioxide waste and cannot pick up oxygen. So, instead of carrying a full quota of life-giving oxygen back to the cells of the body, the bloodstream returns with a mixture of fresh oxygen and a residue of toxic poisons. As this sluggish process continues, the proportion of carbon dioxide buildup increases, causing health problems.

FILL YOUR LUNGS WITH SUPER, LIFE-GIVING OXYGEN

Breath Expansion Test: Before you begin your Bragg Super Power Breathing Program, perform this simple test. Exhale fully and measure your deflated chest with a tape measure. Take a deep breath and measure again. After a month of practicing these exercises, take this test again. You will be amazed by how much more super, life-giving oxygen fills your lungs as you practice Bragg Super Power Breathing.

11

Shallow Breathers Self-Poison Themselves

When you are a shallow breather, you don't change the air at the base of your lungs, where two-thirds of your lung capacity is located. When you return impure blood to your body, the ill effects are compounded because your blood cannot perform properly. It is difficult for blood that is loaded with poisonous wastes to transport the relatively small amount of oxygen which it absorbs; it is even harder for it to carry the necessary nourishment from food. An inadequate oxygen supply impairs your body's ability to break down food into digestible elements. This slows all bodily function. This is why deep breathing is so important for health!

With wrong diet and shallow breathing the organs of elimination are overworked and underfed! But the accumulating wastes must go somewhere. Some are discharged into the sweat glands. This toxic overload produces unpleasant body odors. Other toxic wastes end up deposited as heavy mucus into the sinus cavities, lungs and bronchial tubes. Some line the passages of the ears, eyes, nose and throat, as well as along the digestive tract. Deposits of hardened wastes in the moveable joints can cause pressure on nerves, creating painful warning signals. Pain is Mother Nature's flashing red warning signal that something is wrong in your body. This pain warning should be respected with corrective measures taken right away – not repressed by painkilling drugs full of both known and unknown side effects!

Shallow breathers actually poison themselves by robbing their bodies of sufficient oxygen! This is auto-intoxication (self-poisoning). They are slowly suffocating and dying in their own body wastes and poisons. Pneumonia is a good example; the body and lungs fill up and drown in their own toxins and mucus.

Consider this: if someone deliberately tried to force you to kill yourself by taking shallow breaths, what would you do? You'd fight back! In defiance, you would breathe deeply, cleansing your blood and entire system to give your body more life, energy and super health!

Start practicing Bragg Super Power Breathing Now!

Chapter 3

The Way You Breathe Affects Your Life

When You Breathe Deeply and Fully You Live Longer and More Healthy

When you pump a generous flow of oxygen into your body, every cell becomes more alive! This enables the four main *motors* of your body – the heart, lungs, liver and kidneys – to operate and perform better. Your miracle-working bloodstream purifies and cleanses every part of the body, including itself. This eliminates toxic wastes as Mother Nature planned and fuel (food) and vital oxygen are carried to every cell in your body.

With ample oxygen your muscles, tendons and joints function more smoothly. Your skin becomes firmer and more resilient and your complexion clearer and glowing. You will radiate with greater health and well-being!

With Super Power Breathing your brain becomes more alert and your nervous system functions better. You become free from tension and strain because you can easily take the stresses and pressures of daily living. Your emotions come under your control. You feel joyous and exuberant. If negative emotions such as anger, hate, jealousy, greed or fear intrude, expel them with positive thinking and slow, concentrated deep breathing.

The deep breather enjoys more peace of mind, tranquility and serenity. In India, the great teachers practice deep, full breathing as the first essential step towards higher spiritual development. You attain higher concentration in meditation by taking long, slow, deep breaths. Deep breathing stimulates your brain cells and promotes new brain cell growth, as shown on next page.

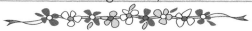

Oxygen is the vital, precious, invisible staff of life. – Paul C. Bragg

13

Super Deep Breathing Improves Your Brain

The person who breathes deeply and fully thinks more clearly and sharply. Oxygen stimulates your logic and intelligence. The more deeply and fully you breathe, the greater your power of concentration and the more your creative mind will assert itself. You will also develop greater extrasensory perception within your body, especially the brain. Scientists at the Salk Institute for Biological Studies, La Jolla, CA, now know that adults do generate new brain cells in the hippocampus, an area in the brain which is responsible for learning and memory. Deep breathing nourishes and fine-tunes the brain and entire body!

Bragg Super Power Breathing will help to constantly rejuvenate you to a higher energy vibration of living! The more fully and deeply you breathe, the further you will travel to higher levels on the physical, mental and spiritual planes. Now close your eyes. Relax a few minutes while doing some slow deep breathing!

Give Thanks to Your Miracle-Working Lungs

Every living thing breathes. Plants breathe through pores in their leaves. In the marvelous balance of Mother Nature, plants breathe in carbon dioxide and give off vital oxygen – while animals inhale oxygen and exhale carbon dioxide. Both thrive in a healthy, natural balance.

Unfortunately humans have played havoc with this natural balance by destroying forests and covering grass with pavement. They continue to poison our already over-burdened air with pollutants from motorized traffic and heavy industry. Wildlife, when it has survived slaughter by man, suffocates in such polluted air. Fish die in polluted waters. How long can people survive in the midst of the environmental poisons which they continually create? This is a question of great concern to us. Read the classic book *Silent Spring* by our friend Rachel Carson, available in most libraries. If followed, her wise advice would have saved America and nations worldwide billions of dollars! We desperately need more courageous and dedicated people like Rachel Carson to show the world the error of its ways!

The Lower Respiratory System

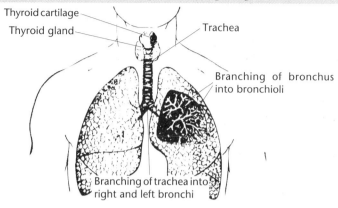

Thyroid cartilage
Thyroid gland
Trachea
Branching of bronchus into bronchioli
Branching of trachea into right and left bronchi

Path of Breath

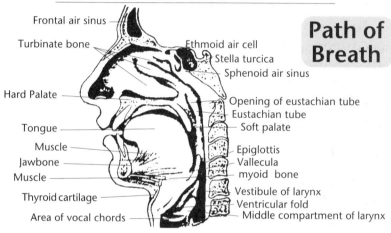

Frontal air sinus
Turbinate bone
Ethmoid air cell
Stella turcica
Sphenoid air sinus
Hard Palate
Opening of eustachian tube
Eustachian tube
Soft palate
Tongue
Muscle
Epiglottis
Jawbone
Vallecula
Muscle
myoid bone
Thyroid cartilage
Vestibule of larynx
Ventricular fold
Area of vocal chords
Middle compartment of larynx

Mechanics of Breathing

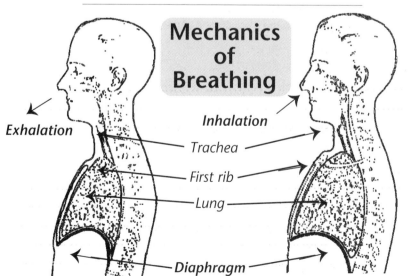

Exhalation

Inhalation
Trachea
First rib
Lung

Diaphragm

The mechanics of breathing, showing the position of the diaphragm and ribs at exhalation and at inhalation

15

The Lungs Are Nature's Miracle Breathers

Every animal extracts oxygen from the environment in which it lives. Through their gills, fish extract oxygen from water (H_2O). Insects get oxygen from the air through alveoli or air cells in individual openings set in segments of their bodies. Worms and other invertebrates breathe through the pores of their skin.

Vertebrate animals, including the human race, have those miracle mechanisms – the lungs. The mechanical equivalent would be a pair of bellows, though the lungs are far more intricate and adaptable.

Human lungs are a miracle pair of conical-shaped organs composed of spongy, porous tissue. They occupy the thoracic cavity (chest) with the heart in the center, and are protected by the amazingly strong and resilient rib cage. The apex of each lung reaches just above the collar bone; the base extends to the waistline.

What makes up our lungs? About 800 million alveoli – air cells or sacs of elastic tissue – which can expand or contract like tiny balloons. If these little air sacs were flattened out and laid side by side, the flattened alveoli would cover an area of 100 square yards!

Tiny capillaries (blood vessels) thread the elastic walls of each of the millions of air sacs . . . and it is through these that the blood passes to discharge its load of poisonous carbon dioxide and absorb the vital, life-giving oxygen. The average person has five to six quarts of blood, which must be cleansed continually.

Air inhaled through the nose and mouth reaches the alveoli through an intricate system of tubes, beginning with the large trachea, or windpipe, which is kept rigid by rings of cartilage in its walls. The trachea extends through the neck into the chest where it divides into two branches (bronchi), each leading into a lung cavity. Each bronchus divides into a number of successively smaller branches to bring air to every air sac.

Breathing is the first place, not the last, one should look when fatigue, disease or other evidence of disordered energy presents itself.
– Dr. Sheldon Hendler, *Author of The Oxygen Breakthrough (amazon.com)*

You Have Lungs – Fill Them Up

Each lung sits perfectly enveloped in a protective elastic membrane, the pleura, whose inner layer is attached to the lung and whose outer layer forms the lining of the thoracic cavity inside the rib cage. One end of each rib is attached to the spinal column, but the front of the rib cage is open. This allows the lungs to expand and contract. When you breathe deeply, filling every air sac, your thoracic cavity expands as your lungs fill with six to ten pints of air. This varies according to body build and size. Lungs occupy from 200 to over 300 cubic inches.

This marvelous breathing mechanism is yours for free! You are born with it. It functions without conscious effort, yet without it, you cannot exist. **Start slow, deep relaxed breathing right now.**

Not even the latest medical inventions used by hospitals in emergencies, however ingenious, can equal your human breathing machine. Perhaps if human beings had to pay a fabulous price for their lungs and air, they would use them to full capacity all the time. Think of the big price you pay for only using them partially by shallow breathing. Remember, we are always only one breath away from death!

The Importance of Clean Air to Health

It is essential to breathe clean air – air that's as free as possible from such chemicals as smog, car exhaust, natural gas appliance fumes and many other toxic chemical pollutants. Our air also needs to be as free as possible from dust, dust mites and their fecal matter, mold, animal dander and pollen. Everyone's health is helped in varying degrees by clean air. It is vitally important to live and work in an area which has clean air and which is free of all harmful fumes. It is also equally important to keep our homes pure, clean and free from dust, dust mites and debris! Most people cannot be truly 100% healthy and well until they breathe clean air, maintain a healthy diet and live a healthy lifestyle.

On an average day your lungs move enough air in and out to fill a medium-sized room or blow up several thousand party balloons.

Live Longer Breathing Clean Air Deeply

We advise those who live, work, etc. in smog-ridden, polluted cities to obtain a good air filter. We especially recommend filters which contain charcoal and a high efficiency particulate HEPA air filter. The charcoal removes most of the chemicals and the HEPA filter removes most of the particles. To be effective in an average room, the flow rate through the filter should be over 200 cubic feet of air per minute. The wise motorist will also install an air filter in his car for cleaning the air while driving in air-polluted cities. Auto stores and catalogs usually stock them.

When we are born, our lungs are new, fresh, clean, and rosy in color. If we could live in a dust-free atmosphere breathing deeply all our lives, then our lungs would remain *as good as new* for a long, healthy lifetime of use. Yet most people abuse their lungs! Some of this comes from external causes. <u>The lungs are the only organs of the body which are directly affected by external conditions, specifically, the air we breathe into them</u>!

Mother Nature has provided protection against a normal amount of dust contamination: tiny hairs in the nose serve as filters and moist mucus in the passages leading to the lungs traps dust particles that we expel through the nose or mouth. The tonsils also serve as guards to trap germs. The lungs protect themselves remarkably well by expelling carbon dioxide through oxygenation and by discharging toxins into the blood for elimination via the kidneys. *Your body is a miracle!*

Unfortunately, most civilized people today live in very unnatural conditions. Almost everywhere there are abnormal amounts of pollutants in the air we breathe, especially in urban areas. Our lungs are often overloaded with more contaminants than they can handle. These are passed along into the bloodstream and to other parts of the body. The lungs of a modern city dweller become brownish from car smog, soot, etc. Even in most farming areas, the lungs must contend with pollens, excessive dust, poisonous pesticides, fertilizers and other toxic chemicals.

A California study shows over 275 people die yearly in smog-riddled L.A. areas from smog. They estimate soon this figure could triple (see pages 92-95 and 122).

Chapter 4

Smoking – A Deadly Habit That Destroys Lungs and Health

With all these nearly inescapable health hazards, smog, etc, in the world to overcome, it's incredible that millions of people harm their lungs even more by inhaling deadly tobacco smoke into their lungs.

Nicotine is poison! It immediately affects lung function and constricts your cardiovascular system. It destroys vitamin C, which is vital to your health and immune system. After only 12 hours of not smoking, nicotine blood levels fall and the heart and lungs begin healing. If you smoke, please stop now and be loving to your body. (Copy pages 19-24, and give to smokers.)

The lungs' air sacs are further damaged by tobacco tars and carbon particles. These lodge in the walls of the lungs' important balloon-like cells, causing them to lose their natural elasticity and eventually breaking them down altogether. The result? **Emphysema** – the killer disease in which destruction of the breathing mechanism slowly smothers its victim from within.

Of the over 50 million Americans who smoke, one third to one half will die from smoking-related diseases! Smoking also introduces at least two deadly poisons into the body: *arsenic* and *carbon monoxide,* as well as other toxins. Compounding these health hazards, smoking creates a desire for caffeine and sugar. Moreover, twice as many smokers drink alcohol compared to non-smokers. Smokers have a far greater incidence of cancer of the lungs, larynx, pharynx, esophagus, mouth, colon and breast. All tobacco products should be banned – they are killers!

If you insist on committing a slow suicide by smoking, no one can stop you. If you really want to save your lungs, health and life, stop smoking by using your strong will and persistence. Start today to make the effort to stop as a positive step towards living The Bragg Healthy Lifestyle.

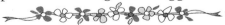

In China smoking is epidemic! Studies show that one-third of the Chinese men will die of tobacco related diseases.

19

Stop Smoking – Save Your Lungs and Life

In our Bragg Health Crusade Lectures throughout the world, we have had thousands of health students who were smokers; some for as long as 40 years. We inspired them to stop smoking and take charge of their health. You can too! Smokers should read about the deadly effects of smoking to the heart and overall health in our book, *Healthy Heart: Keep Your Cardiovascular System Healthy and Fit at Any Age.*

Here's a tip from a writer friend of ours who, over the years, had acquired the habit of lighting a cigarette whenever she paused to compose her next sequence of thoughts. She said, "When it dawned on me what I was doing, I felt like a complete fool. I stopped smoking! It was destroying my health. Now, instead of a cigarette, I take a full, deep breath and I'm healthier and my thoughts come faster and more clearly than ever!"

She finally realized that she did this because her brain was calling for more oxygen. What she actually needed and wanted was a deep breath – but she was inhaling smoke instead of oxygen, thus defeating her purpose.

If you are a smoker, try this! When you want to smoke a cigarette or cigar or pipe – stop! Instead, <u>take a long, slow, deep breath – filling every air sac in your lungs – and hold it, allowing your red blood cells to become more oxygenated – then exhale slowly and completely. Empty every bit of poisonous carbon dioxide from your lungs.</u> You will feel a new surge of energy from the top of your scalp to the soles of your feet . . . a relaxing and incredibly rejuvenating sensation which you can never get from using tobacco or any other artificial stimulant. The surest way to quit a bad habit is to replace it with a good one. . .

The greatest benefit to your life and health would be to replace smoking with deep breathing!

Smoking is Robbing Millions of their Sight

Long-term smokers have over double the risk of developing macular degeneration than nonsmokers. Over 13 million Americans have this and <u>it's the leading cause of vision loss</u>. Boston Researchers speculate that smoking's blinding effects of macular degeneration may be due to a reduction in vital blood flow to the retina, as well as low levels of healthy antioxidants in the body. – AMA Journal

Teens Talk About Stopping Smoking

Ex-smoking teens testify that their life is better, self-esteem higher and hope and joy for the future more profound after they quit smoking! Often these misguided, unfortunate children begin smoking before they are old enough to appreciate their hard-working lungs. They begin filling their miracle breathing lungs with health destroying tobacco, some when they are 16, 14 and even 10 years old! Stan B. recalls, "I started smoking when I was 12, to look cool." Susan W. says, "I smoked 2 packs a day from the time I was 16."

As horrifying as these stories are, we can take heart from these youngsters and learn a lesson from their resiliency. Though they are young and the challenge they face is difficult, many teen smokers are winning the battle against the smoking habit – and feeling healthier and happier as a result! When it comes to quitting, Stan B. admits, "It's not easy, but I look at my parents who've smoked for over 20 years! I know I don't want to be sucking smoke into my lungs and coughing like them."

Every smoking teen should remember that they are not alone in the struggle to quit, and that their goal is within reach. Many young adults now choose a healthy quality of life over one of the greatest destroyers of our time – smoking! And, should any smoking teens find themselves wavering in their efforts to quit, they should remember the words of ex-smoking teen Ann S., who explains, "The biggest reward was that my self-esteem became so much better – I don't need a cigarette to make everything okay. I have made positive changes, enjoy a healthy lifestyle and have more money, time and energy!"

All Tobacco Should Be Banned – it's a Killer!

Shocking Sad Facts: Children and teenagers make up 90% of the new smokers in the United States. Teenage and college smoking is on the rise!

The Teenage Self-Destruction Craze – Smoking, Alcohol & Pot

These are "gateway" habits that can lead to harder drugs and other very dangerous activities. Over 60% of the children who smoke pot before the age of 15 move into the deadly drugs: cocaine, heroin, hallucinogens, etc.

The future depends on what we do in the present. – Gandhi

21

Quit Smoking – See the Difference it Makes!

- **20 MINUTES AFTER QUITTING:** Your blood pressure and pulse rate drop to normal. The temperature of our hands and feet increases to normal.

- **8 HOURS AFTER QUITTING:** The carbon monoxide level in our blood drops to normal. The oxygen level in your blood increases to normal.

- **24 HOURS AFTER QUITTING:** Your chance for heart attack decreases.

- **48 HOURS AFTER QUITTING:** Your ability to taste and smell is enhanced.

- **2 WEEKS TO 3 MONTHS AFTER QUITTING:** Your circulation improves. Walking becomes easier. Your lung function increases as much as 30 percent.

- **1 TO 9 MONTHS AFTER QUITTING:** Coughing, sinus congestion, fatigue and shortness of breath decrease. Your lungs and body are cleaner and more resistant to infection.

- **1 YEAR AFTER QUITTING:** Excess risk for coronary heart disease decreases to 50% that of a smoker's.

- **2 TO 3 YEARS AFTER QUITTING:** The risk for coronary heart disease and stroke decrease compared to those of people who have never smoked. Also less chance of osteoporosis.

- **5 YEARS AFTER QUITTING:** Lung cancer death rate for the former one-pack-per-day smoker decreases by almost half. Risks of mouth and throat cancer are half those of smokers.

- **10 TO 15 YEARS AFTER QUITTING:** Lung cancer death rate is almost that of non-smokers. Pre-cancerous cells are replaced. Risks for mouth, throat, esophagus, bladder, kidney and pancreas cancer decrease. – Prevention Magazine

Fast Return To Health When You Stop Smoking

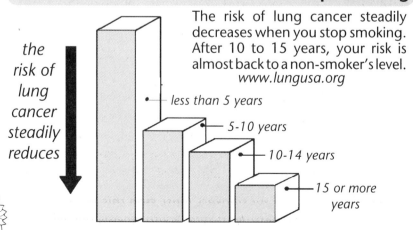

the risk of lung cancer steadily reduces

The risk of lung cancer steadily decreases when you stop smoking. After 10 to 15 years, your risk is almost back to a non-smoker's level.
www.lungusa.org

less than 5 years

5-10 years

10-14 years

15 or more years

DEADLY SMOKING FACTS!

✝ Tobacco use and also second-hand smoke will eventually kill over one fifth of the population now living in the developed world: about 250 million people.

✝ Of the 50 million Americans who smoke, one third to one half will die from a smoke-related disease and all will reduce their life expectancy by an average of nine years.

✝ Smoking acts as either a stimulant or a depressant – depending upon the smoker's emotional state.

✝ The average pack-a-day smoker takes about 70,000 *hits* of nicotine each year. *www.ash.org*

✝ "Second hand smoke" hurts non-smokers: it speeds up the heart rate, raises blood pressure and doubles the amount of deadly carbon monoxide in their blood.

✝ Secondary smoke contains more nicotine, tar and cadmium (leading to hypertension, bronchitis and emphysema) than mainstream smoke.

✝ Babies born to mothers who smoke tend to have lower body weight, smaller lungs and poor health.

✝ Lung illnesses are twice as common in smokers' children.

✝ Children and teenagers make up 90% of the new smokers in the United States – and teenage smoking is on the rise!

✝ The death rate from breast cancer ranges from 25% to 75% higher among women who smoke. *www.breastcancer.org*

✝ Female smokers may face a higher risk of lung cancer – as much as twice the risk of male smokers, according to a study done by Dr. Harvey Risch at Yale University.

✝ Your body contains almost 100,000 miles of blood vessels. Smoking ages & constricts those vessels, depriving your body of important, rich oxygen it needs, this lack causes illness.

✝ Tobacco is the main introduction to more deadly drugs!!!

✝ Teens who smoke are far more likely to engage in other risky and life-threatening behaviors (including using other dangerous drugs; violence; gang involvement; carrying weapons; and engaging in premarital sex which often results in pregnancy or disease) than non-smoking teens.

✝ Cataracts, cancer, angina, arteriosclerosis, osteoporosis, chronic bronchitis, high blood pressure, impotence and respiratory ailments are linked to all forms of smoking.

QUIT SMOKING! All smokers must stop this vicious, deadly habit that destroys health, youth, energy and life.

Health Hazard to Avoid – Deadly Smoking
What it Does to You and Those Around You

When people inhale deadly tobacco smoke into their miracle lungs, the protective cilia hairs filter out much of the smoke's harmful substances before it is exhaled. This means that while harmful toxins are trapped in the delicate linings of the smokers' lungs, fewer of these toxins are re-released into the air for others to breathe in. However, between a smoker's deadly puffs, the cigarette burns directly into the air. This smoke is known as "secondhand, side-stream" smoke, but it should be called "direct" smoke. Smoke that burns directly into the air is completely unfiltered and more deadly than the smokers' smoke! Stay away from all deadly smoke!

Recent studies establish that people who live or work around smokers are more likely to develop lung and sinus damage than smokers. For asthma or bronchitis sufferers, this exposure is very damaging. In addition to these dangers, "direct" smoke irritates the eyes, nose and throat and smells up everything it touches (rooms, hotels, offices, carpets, drapes, cars and everything around smoking).

For the cigarette smoker, whose miracle lungs have unfortunately become the filters protecting the body from the deadly smoke, the effects are equally – if not more – damaging. Tar begins to collect in the lungs once there is too much to be removed through the lungs' normal cleaning processes. This means the over-burdened lungs can no longer clean normal contaminants they have to deal with. Dirt inhaled into the alveoli – which is normally trapped in a layer of sticky mucus and carried out of the lungs by the wavelike motions of the tiny cilia hairs – becomes trapped and stuck in the lungs. The cilia hairs become paralyzed by tar, so the normal cleansing (drain) procedures break down and the airways become clogged. This makes the lungs resort to coughing, spitting and respiratory-breathing attacks, flu, etc. in an effort to expel the contaminated, clogging toxins, tar and mucus.

There is good news. When a person stops smoking the cilia hairs begin to heal and move again. Smokers – stop now and begin cleansing and healing immediately!

24

Chapter 5

Common Cold – The Body's Miracle Cleansing Process

Any one day in winter, over 30 million Americans suffer with a bad cold. Adults average five to six colds per season, while children and teenagers often get double that amount. The body wants the toxins out!

Are these colds necessary? How do people *catch cold?* What causes the common cold? Medical Science has learned how to control many diseases that are far more serious, but remains baffled by the common cold. Is the culprit an unfiltered virus? Is it brought on by sitting in a draft, getting chilled, or getting one's feet wet, as is often suggested by mothers through the ages?

Colds Clean Out Mucus and Toxins

While the theories are many, there seems to be only one sure fact – people who are in perfect health don't *catch colds.* My dad spent a year living in the Arctic among the Eskimos. He never had a cold, and neither did they. He had the same experience in the South Seas, in the Balkans, among the nomads of the Middle East and with the native tribes of Africa. The common factor among all these people is that they breathe pure air, eat simple natural foods and get plenty of exercise and sleep. By following this same basic healthy lifestyle, my Dad remained free of colds even in the midst of civilization.

Based on his research, he found that the *common cold* is Mother Nature's and God's method of detoxifying the body. Most people are shallow breathers. And most live on an unhealthy diet of devitalized foods. Toxins start accumulating and clogging their bodies. That's why it's important to live a healthy lifestyle, plus some fasting.

When you feel a cold or any illness coming on, or are just depressed – it is best to fast! Each time you fast, you will feel better. Your body will then have a chance to heal and rebuild its immune system by regular fasting.
– James Balch, M.D., Co-Author, *Prescription for Nutritional Healing*
"Bragg books were my conversion to the healthy way."

25

The Body Self-Cleanses, Repairs & Heals

When the toxicity of these accumulated poisons, mucus, etc., exceeds the body's tolerance, the natural vital forces set up a miracle *cleansing-healing* (common colds) crisis. The body induces a rise in body temperature (fever) to burn up the many toxins, while others are eliminated by a heavy discharge of mucus from the nose, mouth and throat. If the toxic overload is heavy, there may be a discharge of mucus from the bowels and perhaps diarrhea.

Instead of being alarmed, be grateful that your body's natural Vital Forces are strong enough to take command and get rid of the toxins that you have accumulated! Don't try to block this natural healing process with antibiotics. Work with Mother Nature. Breathe deeply and fully to supply your body with the great purifier: oxygen. Rest and fast (page 114). Do a distilled water (8 glasses daily) fast or try a fresh juice fast (page 117). It is best to take only liquids during this cleansing and healing crisis. Your amazing body will fight for its life against a great deal of abuse. When you follow Mother Nature's and God's Laws and live The Bragg Healthy Lifestyle you can create a painless, tireless and ageless body. Miracles can happen!

Colds and Oxygen are Great Cleansers

If you *catch cold,* remember you are passing through a natural cleansing and healing crisis. Heed the warning – fast! Mother Nature is telling you: *You have allowed your body to become poisoned with toxic wastes and maybe by overeating. Work with me now by fasting – to cleanse your body of these toxins. Once this cleansing crisis has passed, now keep your body clean by following my Laws of Natural Living!*

Often people tell us that they have a bad case of the *flu.* When we ask where they got it, this is what we hear – *The flu's going around. Everyone's got it."* We then ask, *Where can we find it? We'd like to meet some flu germs!* They stare at us in utter amazement. To help them out of their mental confusion, we explain that when you breathe fully, live a healthy lifestyle and eat natural foods, free from all refining, processing and chemical additives – it's then that you can build a powerful immunity against germs, viruses and illness!

Oxygen Cleanses and Nourishes

No germ can live in freshly squeezed organic orange juice because there is nothing in pure orange juice for it to feed on. All germs, regardless of their names, are scavengers! They feed on toxic decaying matter.

It's our personal opinion, based on experience and research, that a 100% healthy, natural foods diet – in combination with the enormous amount of pure oxygen pumped into the body by the vigorous breathing exercises taught in this book – help provide a natural immunity against most infectious diseases and germs.

Oxygen is not only the energizing factor which makes it possible for the body to eliminate the putrefied matter on which germs thrive, it also exterminates the germs. As you breathe deep more oxygen into your body and nourish it with organic, healthy foods, you give your body a greater ability to ward off germs and infections!

When we practice Super Power Breathing, we increase our cardiovascular respiratory power. We purify and energize our bloodstream to carry more powerful, revitalizing oxygen to the heart and entire cardiovascular system. Start today – you will benefit greatly.

Breathing is our connection to life, through the body and heart, leading us to a wholeness of being and giving us spirit for living life to its fullest. – S. Hainer, M.S.

It never hurts to brush up on the 3 Rs:

- *Respect for yourself.*   • *Respect towards others.*
- *Responsible living today, tomorrow and always!*

Start Being Happier, Smile & Laugh More – It's Up To You!

Healthy actions speak louder than words and can elevate your mood if you feel depressed. Take a brisk walk in a natural setting and practice slow, deep breathing – it helps you sort out and solve problems. Spend time with children, it simplifies life and puts everything in perspective. Find the comics in the newspaper or something funny to read and laugh. If someone is upset, try to analyze the situation from that person's perspective. As often as possible make yourself smile and laugh; it opens the blood vessels in the back of your head to physically lift your mood. Choose to be happy in spite of circumstances. No one "makes" you happy – it's an inner attitude that sparkles from within.

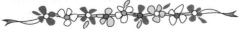

Laughter is inner jogging, and good for your body and soul. – Norman Cousins

WE THANK THEE

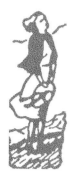

For flowers that bloom about our feet;
   For song of bird and hum of bee;
For all things fair we hear or see,
   Father in heaven we thank Thee!
For blue of stream and blue of sky;
   For pleasant shade of branches high;
For fragrant air and cooling breeze;
   For beauty of the blooming trees;
Father in heaven we thank Thee!
   For mother love and father care,
For brothers strong and sisters fair;
   For love at home and here each day;
For guidance lest we go astray,
   Father in heaven we thank Thee!
For this new morning with its light;
   For rest and shelter of the night;
For health and food, for love and friends;
   For every thing His goodness sends,
Father in heaven we thank Thee!
   – Ralph Waldo Emerson

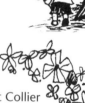

Doubt destroys. Faith builds! – Robert Collier

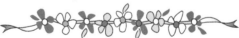

A healthy body is a guest-chamber for the soul;
a sick body is a prison. – Francis Bacon

The law, "Whatsoever a man sows that he shall also reap," is
inscribed in flaming letters upon the portal of Eternity, and none can deny it,
none can cheat it and none can escape it. – James Allen

Progress is impossible without change, and those who cannot change
their minds cannot change anything. – George Bernard Shaw

Self-discipline is your golden key; without it, you cannot be happy.
– Maxwell Maltz, M.D. – Bragg follower we greatly admired.

The unexamined life is not worth living. It is time to
re-evaluate your past as a guide to your future. – Socrates

A bird does not fly because it has wings; it has wings because it flies.
– Robert Ardney

Chapter 6

Your Miracle Nose – Pathway to the Lungs

The Bragg Super Power Breathing technique is the most essential part of The Bragg Healthy Lifestyle. Your nose and nasal passageways are essential factors in all your breathing. So it's important that we understand the nose and the vital role it plays in breathing.

The nose is a system of passages and hollow spaces that link the external nose to the eyes, ears, mouth and throat. It is through this intricate pathway that oxygen-rich air travels from our nose to our lungs. You might wonder why we have all this complicated breathing mechanism made up of cartilage, bone, and soft tissue organized into several pairs of hollow air-spaces called sinuses. When afflicted with some sinus or nasal complaint you might think it just can't be worth all the trouble. After all, the mouth and throat seem to do the breathing work just fine — and it's just a simple and direct air pathway to the lungs.

We Mostly Breathe Through the Nose

We do most breathing through the nose. That means that the oxygen required to nourish our bodies moves through the nose between 30,000 to 60,000 times a day, depending upon whether you are a shallow, deep or slow breather. So then, why is this part of our body so complex and a site of so many health complaints? The answer is that the nose is a lot more than just a pathway for air to get to the lungs, it's a miracle working part of your body.

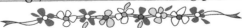

Shallow breathing helps to increase symptoms of almost every known sickness!

A large percent of sinus problems are caused by bacteria, smoke, diet (milk, etc.).

The quality of the blood depends largely upon its oxygenation in the lungs.
– Basic Physiology

When we begin to trust ourselves more, the body begins to renew itself and becomes healthier and filled with more life energy. – Shakti Gawain

Your Nose is a Miracle Air-Filtration System

The hollow spaces of the nose - called sinuses - act as "echo chambers" (*eight air pockets*), which make our voices resonate (unless sinuses are stuffed up). These open spaces (located behind our eyebrows, nose, cheeks, and between the eyes) also give us better balance and cushion the brain from blows to the head. Our sense of smell is located in the nose. The most important function of the nose, the sinuses and nose hairs, is to condition and filter the air as it passes through to your faithful, hard-working lungs.

The membranes of the nose and sinuses produce between a pint and a quart of mucus every day. These secretions line the walls of the nose and sinuses and are always on the move. As the mucus passes through the sinus cavities, it collects dust particles, bacteria and other air pollutants that were breathed in along with the oxygen-rich air that nourishes every corner of the body. These same airways are lined with little filter hairs (called *cilia*) which strongly try to keep out all dust and pollutants from the air we breathe.

As you can see, God entrusts some very important duties to the nose. It's the nose that tries its best to protect the lungs and all your body cells from any airborne pollutants and contaminants. Under healthy conditions, our lungs receive clean air even with some pollution, thanks to our nose filters! Sadly, in the world many areas have heavy pollution that plagues our air and takes its toll on the health of the body! The nose takes the brunt of the attack, then lungs and the body.

Sinusitis Causes Breathing Infection Problems

Sinus complaints usually are signs of the nose trying to do its job of protecting the lungs in troubled times. The nasal passages can suffer from the contaminants they work hard to block. Sometimes the sinuses become irritated or inflamed from air pollution, smoke, mold, pet dander, infection, or an allergy (milk, etc) attack brought on by some of these irritating toxic factors.

The body is self-cleansing and self-healing when you give it a chance with a fasting detox cleanse and living a healthy lifestyle! – Patricia Bragg

Blocked Sinuses Breed Health Problems

When the nose and sinuses become over-burdened, they secrete mucus and swell. This blocks the openings and prevents the free flow of mucus and air. This causes a breathing problem that creates an environment where bacteria can flourish. This unhealthy situation weakens the nose and sets the stage for sinus and asthma problems, poor breathing, mucus plugged sinuses and infections, etc.

Many people who suffer from blocked and painful sinuses run to the drug store for over-the-counter medical relief. Forcing the sinuses open continually can cause harm, because they close up to protect the lungs from airborne toxins, etc. "Temporarily, nasal decongestants and nose drops may give some relief," says Joel R. Saper, M.D., Director of the Michigan Headache Institute. "But if your sinuses are the problem, longer use puts you at risk for a chronic situation of diminishing returns." Instead of the quick-fix relief of a drug, take a long-term view of your nose's health. Remember, your nose is the pathway to your lungs, and the point of entry for the body's most needed, elemental nutrient – oxygen. Your nose deserves to be treated with loving, gentle care.

Nasal Wash & Herbs Bring Relief & Healing

In addition to healthy living and avoiding dairy, you can relieve symptoms of sinusitis and bolster your nose health with this nasal wash: Add ½ tsp Bragg Organic Apple Cider Vinegar to cup of warm distilled water, to help clean out mucus and any infection. (*You can alternate using ½ tsp celtic salt.*) This wash helps mucus membranes and sinuses to better dispose of any pollutants in your air. Cup liquid in hand or use squeeze spray bottle; sniff up right nostril, roll head back, then side to side, lean over, blow out mucus. Then repeat with other side. Do twice daily until mucus subsides. Herbs(teas or caps - fenugreek, echinacea, anise, marshmallow and red clover) help to loosen phlegm and clear congestion; rosehips, horehound and mullein help relieve symptoms. Most importantly, drink 8 or more glasses of distilled water daily. Add Bragg Organic Vinegar to 3 of them. (*See recipe page 116.*)

One physician told medical students to be leary of all new drug research.
– Sandra Tanenbaum, Hospital & Health Services, Professor Ohio State University

31

Solve Sinus and Allergy Problems

For a healthy nose, it's essential you live The Bragg Healthy Lifestyle. A balanced, healthy life is the basis for your good health! A healthy, happy head and body are necessary preconditions to a healthy nose. If you live in a polluted area, or if your sinuses are already damaged from the hard work of protecting your lungs, buy a high-efficiency HEPA (microscopic pores remove almost all particles) air filtration system. This pre-filters and cleans the air you breathe, making the job easier for your nose. Also enjoy the herbal teas on page 31 or take them in capsule form. <u>Inhalation of eucalyptus, basil, lavender, and peppermint oils help blocked sinuses. Put a few drops into boiling water, turn heat off, and then carefully breathe the vapors.</u>

You must be intelligent about allergies. If you know you're allergic to particular substances, take precautions to avoid them. If you suspect allergies, take all necessary steps to learn if and what you are allergic to. (Do test on page 33.) The most common allergens are mold spores, animal dandruff, and house dust. Also, food allergies (below) are high sources of allergic reactions; they are associated with the nose, sinus, and mucus complaints.

<u>It is of utmost importance to avoid dairy products.</u> Millions suffer allergic reactions (mucus, colds, etc.) to dairy products because they are very unhealthy for the nose and the whole body. Dairy proteins can cause the nose and throat airway passages to swell. They also produce mucus-causing sinus discomfort and bacterial conditions. If you snore (pg 81) or suffer a sinus condition, a non-dairy diet brings miracle improvements.

> **Read these 2 important books on milk and why to avoid milk:**
> • Mad Cows and Milk Gate *by Virgil Hulse M.D. (541) 482-2048*
> • Milk, the Deadly Poison *by Robert Cohen (888) 668-6455*
>   *visit websites: www.notmilk.com and www.milkgate.com*

Most Common Food Allergies

- *MILK: Butter, Cheese, Cottage Cheese, Ice Cream, Milk, Yogurt*
- *CEREALS & GRAINS: Wheat, Corn, Buckwheat, Oats, Rye*
- *EGGS: Cakes, Custards, Dressings, Mayonnaise, Noodles*
- *FISH: Shellfish, Crabs, Lobster, Shrimp, Shadroe*
- *MEATS: Bacon, Chicken, Pork, Sausage, Veal, Smoked Products*
- *FRUITS: Citrus Fruits, Melons, Strawberries*
- *NUTS: Peanuts, Pecans, Walnuts, chemically dried, preserved nuts*
- *MISCELLANEOUS: Chocolate, China Black Tea, Cocoa, Coffee, MSG, Palm and Cottonseed Oils, Salt, Spices and allergic reactions often caused by toxic pesticides on salad greens, vegetables, fruits, etc.*

Nosebleeds

Another common health complaint is nosebleeds. Various conditions cause nosebleeds, including blows to the face, excessive dryness, changes in atmospheric pressure, scratching or blowing the nose too strenuously.

Nosebleeds can be classified either as anterior (discharging out the nose) or posterior (discharging down the throat). Posterior bleeding originates in the sinus cavities behind the eyebrows, nose or between the eyes. No matter what position the person is in, the blood will drain out the back of the mouth and down the throat. This condition can affect the elderly that have high blood pressure and they need their doctor's advice. The anterior nosebleed is common variety and flows out nostrils – although if one lies down, the blood may flow down throat. Rarely serious, it can usually be treated by applying pressure to the nose and ice to the injured area. (Soak cotton ball in Bragg Apple Cider Vinegar, lightly pack in nostril and press – this helps blood to coagulate.)

Take these precautions to prevent nosebleeds. Because excessively dry air can cause nasal membranes to crack, form crusts and bleed, increase the humidity in your house if you reside in a dry climate. You can do this with a commercial humidifier. If you need a quick fix, place a pan of boiling water in a small room. To help alleviate dry, sore nasal membranes gently pat aloe-vera, vit.E, Bragg Organic Olive Oil or comfrey ointment inside your nose.

Nosebleeds might be caused by a vitamin K deficiency. This is a crucial mineral for normal blood clotting. If you don't have your fair share, your nose will be more likely to bleed at the least provocation. You can remedy this situation by practicing wise, healthy, natural eating habits. Best vitamin K sources include sprouts, all dark-green leafy vegetables, sea greens, oats, eggs, molasses, alfalfa, wheatgrass, barley and spirulina, etc.

A Self-Test for Specific Problem Foods

Do a 4-day distilled water fast and most food allergies will clear up. Keep a daily Journal, then allow your usual foods one at a time back into your diet. You will soon find out which foods to eliminate from your diet when problems occur.

Your body suffers when you're water dehydrated. The body's cells are like sponges. It takes time for cells to become hydrated. Daily drink 8 glasses of distilled water.

33

Mind Food for Thought to Share

Freedom and progress rest in man's continual searching for truth.
Truth is the summit of being. – Ralph Waldo Emerson

The nation badly needs to go on a diet. It should do something drastic about excessive, unattractive, life-threatening fat. It should get rid of it in the quickest possible way and this is by fasting. – Allan Cott, M.D.

Young men in their 20s who are 20 pounds or more overweight nearly double their chances of developing osteoarthritis of the knee and hip in latter life, according to a long-term study of graduates from the Johns Hopkins School of Medicine. – UC Berkeley Wellness Letter

---

There are over 15 million allergic people in the United States. About half feel their symptoms are severe enough to warrant professional assistance.
– Dr. William Stuart, Nasal Maintenance

Remember always, you are punished by your bad habits of living,
– sooner or later – Paul C. Bragg, N.D.,Ph.D.,

Negative factors like air, soil and water pollutants, acid rain, UV radiation caused by the depletion of the earth's protective ozone layer, chemically treated foods, the disturbance of immune systems through repeated toxic vaccination and immunization, not to mention our stress-infused lifestyles, result in reduced immune response and the inability of our bodies to cope with or neutralize allergens. – Dr. Linda Page, *Allergy Control and Management*

With improving the body's oxygenation and energy utilization at the cellular level, you are strengthening the immune system which is the bodyguard of your health.

The more natural food you eat, the more you'll enjoy radiant health and be able to promote the higher life of love and brotherhood.
– Patricia Bragg, N.D.,Ph.D.

It's Never Too Late to Start Exercising:

Studies show it is never too late to begin exercising. People who begin exercise programs can benefit from this news even if they didn't exercise in the past. Recent physical activity has a greater positive impact on cardiovascular disease and mortality than exercise done in one's past. The cardiovascular health benefits of recent physical activity are more pronounced than with distant physical activity, even though both are beneficial. A consistent maintenance exercise program produced the best overall results in this recent study!
– Sports Medicine Digest, *www.sportmedicine.com*

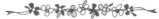

"There is but one way to live and that is Mother Nature's and God's Healthy Way!"

Chapter 7

Unhealthy Buildings Cause Many Breathing and Health Problems

Unhealthy

Healthy

Because we human beings have managed to pollute the water, air, and earth, our Mother Nature suffers. We know now that to stay healthy we must take precautions in some areas when we go in the great outdoors – or even in our backyard. But, it is probably a surprise to most people that even the "great indoors" can be unhealthy and polluted also. Many of our homes and buildings are so toxic that they are unfit to live and work in.

Today unfortunately many of our modern homes and buildings, even cars that shelter and protect us from the elements contain invisible vapors that slowly poison us as they give shelter! Contamination sources are many – and far too unrecognized and unaddressed.

Toxic Building Materials

Toxic building materials are the major source of environmental contaminants inside our homes, schools and places of business. Over the years builders have used many dangerous substances. The evils of **asbestos** are well-known. Other deadly substances include **roofing materials** and **insulation** – especially those made with **formaldehyde**, because they leak poisonous vapors.

Wallpaper and paints are also laden with dangerous chemicals that emit silent poisonous gasses. In addition, the horrors of **lead paint** still threaten many people living in older homes. What about **synthetic carpets**? That soft carpeting that feels cozy to your feet is often a chemical soup which constantly sheds toxic vapors into your home. Crawling toddlers are the most vulnerable.

The preservation of health is a duty. Few seem conscious that there is such a thing as physical morality. – Herbert Spencer

Do not underestimate the dangers posed by **synthetic carpeting**! A Honolulu attorney we knew was slowly paralyzed as a result of the **toxic vapors** given off from his new office carpeting. After several years of litigation, his family finally won a large lawsuit against those responsible for his suffering and death.

Formaldehyde Gives Off Toxic Vapors

Above your head, under your feet, on and in your walls, all around you in your home, formaldehyde could be poisoning your home and you. Many contractors continue to use this toxic chemical as a preservative, binding agent and insulator. It turns up everywhere in our homes and buildings. Despite its widespread use, we know that formaldehyde is an eye, nose, throat and skin irritant – and is a strong suspected carcinogen!

How do you cure your house of formaldehyde sickness? Unfortunately little can be done unless you build your house from scratch with careful attention to using only safe, natural building materials. Beyond this, only time will purify and heal the sick home. Over many years the toxic residues in building materials emit less and less harmful vapors, making the older home a healthier home - and the people who live there become healthier too. Our Santa Barbara home is 90 years old.

Beware of Invisible Radon Dangers

Many factors, some obvious and some not, contribute to the toxic burden of our living and working spaces. Like formaldehyde, radon is an invisible killer lurking in many of our homes and buildings. This odorless, colorless gas is a naturally occurring radioactive by-product given off by stones, soil and water. Radon is a hit or miss threat depending on the land where a home is built. Also all natural stones and bricks used in construction should be checked for radon.

Although not much can be done, it's important to find out if your home is sick from radon contamination. Contact your local health department and ask if you live in a high radon area. If you have any concerns, ask to have a radon test done in your home. Also ask about remedial actions. If your home has high radon levels, seriously consider moving into a healthy home. Radon is the second leading cause of lung cancer after smoking. **Check the web for more radon info:** www.radon.com or http://energy.cr.usgs.gov/radon/radonhome.html. This site will take you to great links on radon dangers.

Healthy Home Environment is Important Check for Lead, Radon, Formaldehyde

Who wants to be sick and live in a sick home? You make the effort to eat well, sleep well and get exercise, don't drop the ball when it comes to ensuring a healthy living environment. **Here's some playing-it-safe ideas:**

First, be sure you and your family are safe from the dangers of **radon**. **Second**, be safe from the dangers of **formaldehyde**; older homes usually have less. Radon contamination is often worse in older homes. **Third**, be safe from the dangers of **lead paint** which is greater in older homes. Test for all three when considering a home. Have a licensed home inspector check for all three toxins and others that might be sickening the home, building, apartment, etc. you live in. It's reasonable and important.

Don't cover floors with **toxic carpeting**. If you must put something on wood floors, carpets and area rugs made from natural materials, wool or cotton are safest. Don't cook with gas in an **unventilated room**. Be sure that your gas flame burns a clean blue. If you cook in a closed room with an orange flame you and your house will suffer from carbon dioxide, carbon monoxide, and other toxins.

To make a safe and healthy home, spend the money to equip your house with plenty of windows and doors Remember what the good doctor said for countless centuries: plenty of clean, fresh air is one of the best cures. Keep your house well ventilated so that there can never be a poisonous buildup of dangerous toxins. Because poisons are often carried around the home by dust particles, it's wise to consider buying a home air purifier that removes these toxic particles.

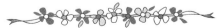

The journey of a thousand miles begins with one step. – Lao Tzu

Having a Healthy, Safe Home and More

Ensuring that your home is a healthy and safe space for you and your family is not an easy task. But what job could be more rewarding than health, happiness, vitality and a long, productive life? Creating a healthy home might not be inexpensive. However the savings in health care costs, lost productivity, worry and stress will greatly outweigh the short-term costs of making your home a safe haven. (Your home should be your health retreat.)

After you've done what you can about toxic walls and vapors, carpets, appliances and the rest, here's a few more suggestions to help reduce your home's toxicity. Read labels of all cleaning products, sprays, etc. in your home. Most are full of toxic ingredients. (Store toxic products in garage.) This includes detergents, soaps, fabric softeners, polishes, upholstery, carpet and oven cleaners, air fresheners, etc. Using toxic household cleansers, fly, ant, bug and moth repellents, etc. exposes people to harmful vapors! Beware of ammonia, turpentine, paint, acetone, chlorine, sodium hydroxide, bleach, gasoline and all toxic vapors.

If you need to use any of these substances, consider only the safe, non-toxic, natural versions. Today most health stores carry complete lines of alternative (healthy) household products, health detergents, etc. Read labels when you shop and buy only healthy alternatives to caustic, toxic chemicals, soaps, toothpastes (*avoid all fluorides*), household cleansers, shampoos and cosmetics, etc. Two healthy substitutes to use for the household cleansers, deodorizers and disinfectants are baking soda and white vinegar (*use for home cleaning, not for recipes*).

Check these websites for healthy, safe products to use:

✔ realgoods.com ✔ ecomart.net ✔ shaklee.com
✔ greenmarketplace.com ✔ ecomall.com
✔ naturaltoys.com ✔ emagazine.com
✔ greenliving.org ✔ greenculture.com

Asthma May Come From Our Environment

Over 14 million Americans experience frightening attacks of wheezing and breathlessness that are sometimes fatal. Asthma is not just one disease. Sometimes it's from an allergy, sometimes it's food related. Asthma may be tied to factors such as what's inside your home, your genes, childhood infections, diet, stress, toxins, etc.

Pollutants may react chemically to the body's tissues. Researchers are looking at many irritants – like latex, which sloughs off automobile tires as tiny particles that may end up in our lungs. Some city studies pinpointed cockroaches as a key allergen. Energy conservation has locked people in sick, "tight" office buildings and homes with sick, stale air, environmental toxins, gas appliances, secondhand smoke, pet hair and dander, mold, bacteria-laden dust and mites.

Treating Asthma Naturally Brings Results!

Famous Dr. Andrew Weil, stated in his Self Healing Letter, "I have seen asthma disappear completely in response to major diet shifts such as eliminating sugar milk products and switching to a healthy vegetarian regime." Johns Hopkins Hospital Studies and others suggest those who monitored their diets, low in meat and additives, were less likely to have asthma problems. Still, most doctors believe erroneously there is no cure for asthma. Asthma attacks can be life-threatening. For short-term acute asthma help, bronchodilating drugs (often addictive with side effects) are at times necessary until breathing improves. There are natural remedies that, while not substitutes for bronchodilators, may help manage acute asthma episodes until breathing improves:

If using inhalers now – try the new medication called Advair Diskus that is giving relief to asthma suffers. Used once daily it works as a preventative instead of an emergency asthma inhaler. For people who use a steroid inhaler 2-3 times per day, this may bring permanent relief from having to use inhalers! We hope those who have breathing problems will soon be so improved like Paul Wenner (pg 5), they will have no need for medication!

Lobelia: Lobelia is used by many naturopathic physicians to treat asthma. Keep on hand a mixture combining three parts tincture of lobelia with one part tincture of capsicum (red pepper). At start of asthmatic attack, take 5 to10 drops of mixture in distilled water. As needed repeat every 30 – 60 minutes up to 4 times for total of three or four doses.

Chinese Ephedra: This famous medicinal plant (Ephedra sinica) is the natural source of ephedrine, a stimulant and bronchodilating agent. You can buy dried ephedra stems from Chinese herb shops and brew them into a pleasant-tasting tea. Put a handful of crumbled stems in a glass or enamel pot of cold water. Bring to a boil, lower heat, cover and boil gently for 20 minutes. Strain. Drink 1 to 2 cups every 2 to 4 hours as needed. (Caution – too much can cause jitteriness and insomnia.)

The Heimlich Maneuver: This versatile maneuver may be life-saving for more than choking victims. The Heimlich Institute is currently teaching asthma patients how to push up on their own diaphragm (more gently than in cases of choking) to help expel trapped air and clear the bronchia of mucus plugs. See page 130 for information on Heimlich.

Self-Health Care for Healthy Lungs

Because standard drugs are suppressive in nature, they tend to perpetuate asthma and reduce the chance that it will disappear on its own – especially in children. Try these natural self-care measures to prevent attacks, improve lungs health and lessen the need for drugs.

● **Use a peak-flow meter,** a hand-held device that you can blow into to measure the amount of air in your lungs.

● **Reduce asthma and respiratory trigger**s by learning causes. Try to eliminate destructive triggers from your life.

● **Drink 8 to 10 glasses of distilled water daily**, to keep respiratory-tract secretions moist and fluid. Drinking plenty of water speeds the process of eliminating irritants and toxins from the body. Avoid dehydration – it causes your body to produce histamine (an asthma-inducing agent) in an effort to prevent water loss through the lungs.

● **Supplement your diet daily with 3,000 mg. vitamin C.**

● **Say "no" to milk and dairy products** which increase secretions of mucus and worsens asthma and allergies!

● **Change your diet.** Food allergies (page 32) trigger many chronic asthma attacks and respiratory-breathing problems.

● **Be manipulated.** Go to a chiropractor or osteopath and have them check for any restrictions in the back, neck, chest and diaphragm areas. A skilled practitioner can free them up. When its needed this can help promote healing.

● **Exercise wisely.** Warm up slowly with stretching and breathing exercises (at least 10 to 15 minutes). Don't jog within 50 feet of a heavy traffic road (car fumes are toxic). Enjoy parks with lawns, trees and fresh clean air.

● **Clear the air.** Use HEPA filters (page 18) in whole room areas or entire house filter system and also use in your car.

● **Hang some plants** (Spider plants, Boston ferns, English Ivy, etc.) in your house, work, office, etc. Plants absorb toxic vapors & gases that help purify the air for your lungs.

● **Relax.** Do breathing exercises and get rest (pages 67-71).

● **Consider healing healthy alternatives** (pages 161-164). Example: a young asthmatic patient was so improved after two months of a Ayurvedic health treatment that he dispensed with most of his medication (pages 44-45).

 Pollutants may negatively react chemically with body's tissues. – Dr. Andrew Weil

Chapter 8

Your Diaphragm – The Key to Bragg Super Power Breathing

What is our secret of deep Super Power Breathing? How can you draw air into the very base of your lungs? Not by merely sniffing it in through your nose nor by gasping it in through your mouth!

Babies breathe naturally by using their diaphragms to create suction which pulls air into the lungs. Air may enter the body through either the nose or the mouth. But the force which draws the air in, filling the air sacs of the lungs to capacity, comes from the strong muscular action of the powerful diaphragm.

The diaphragm is a dome-shaped sheet of strong muscle fibers. It separates the thoracic (upper) half of your body, which contains the heart and lungs – from the abdominal (lower) cavity, which houses the organs of digestion and elimination. The diaphragm stretches from the sternum (breastbone) in front and across the bottom of the ribs to the backbone.

As the diaphragm expands and flattens, it moves downward, producing suction within the chest cavity and pulling air into the lungs (inhalation). When the diaphragm relaxes and rises, it forces air out of the lungs (exhalation). Both operations are equally important: inhalation to bring in life-giving oxygen; exhalation to expel all of the poisonous carbon dioxide.

Exercise and living longer go together! Exercise can be a brisk walk 3 times a week, plus at least 30 – 60 minutes a day of general, constant movement. Even doing such mundane activities as gardening, housework and climbing stairs helps to lower risk for heart disease, claim sports doctors who focus on athletic training. – Sports Medicine Digest

---

The USDA has issued new dietary guidelines encouraging more exercise vegetables & consumption of less fat. The guidelines also stress the use of dietary sources of vitamins & minerals, especially antioxidants & B vitamins, including folic acid. In addition, the guidelines point out that diet is important to health at all stages of life & can help reduce the risk of diseases of all kinds.

41

Diaphragmatic Versus Chest Breathing

Chest breathing results from the movement of the rib section of the trunk, especially the upper section of the chest. When a person inhales, the chest expands, becoming larger. When he exhales, the chest relaxes, becoming smaller. When performed to the limit of inhalation and exhalation, it's an excellent form of internal exercise that helps the whole waist area. It also develops the chest and has many other health benefits.

A great deal is made about *chest expansion . . .* the number of inches which the chest expands from a relaxed position (after exhalation) to that when the lungs are filled with air. However, people with large chests breathe no more effectively than those people with average-sized chests who use their breathing organs efficiently to spread oxygen throughout their bodies.

Chest Breathing: the body undertakes this natural method only during strenuous exertion. It might be termed a form of *forced breathing.* It is an emergency measure. Unfortunately, most people rob themselves of oxygen when they breathe because they use only a minimum of the top portion of their lungs.

Diaphragmatic Breathing: this is the natural method designed for the body. When you inhale, the diaphragm expands. It not only expands the chest cavity and draws air into the lungs, but it also expands the abdominal cavity. It does more than just drawing in air, it stretches and massages the abdominal muscles and organs. When you exhale the diaphragm relaxes. It expels air from the lungs, exercises the rib muscles and massages the heart. Because this tones and tightens the abdominal muscles, you get healthier with each super power breath!

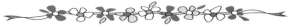

Wake up and say, "Today I am going to be happier, healthier and wiser in my daily living. I am the captain of my life and am going to steer it for 100% healthy lifestyle living!" Fact: Happy people look younger, live longer and have fewer health problems! – Patricia Bragg, N.D., Ph.D.

Nature, time and patience are the 3 greatest physicians. – Irish Proverb

42

The secret of longevity is eating intelligently. – Gaylord Hauser

Internal Massage by Diaphragmatic Action

The diaphragm's effect on the muscles and organs of the abdomen is highly beneficial. To combat the pull of gravity and hold the abdominal organs in place, our abdominal muscles need all the exercise we can find time to give them. Correct, natural diaphragmatic breathing – along with daily exercise and practicing good posture – helps to accomplish many health miracles.

Your diaphragmatic natural action also provides an important massage for the heart, chest and stomach areas, and the liver, intestines, kidneys, gallbladder, spleen and pancreas. This stimulates blood circulation and helps these organs to perform the functions which are essential to maintaining life and health.

The dual action of the diaphragm, which affects the upper thoracic organs (heart and lungs) and the lower abdominal organs, is a vital factor in good blood circulation. This is especially true as blood returns through the veins to the heart. The forceful pumping thrust of the heart muscles sends blood coursing through the arteries. This force is almost spent by the time the bloodstream has dispensed oxygen, nutrients and collected wastes, and is ready to return to the heart through the veins. The return trip is dependent upon the contraction of the muscles and muscular walls of the viscera – the internal organs contained within the abdominal and thoracic cavities. The rhythmic massage of the abdominal organs by the respiratory muscles plays a pivotal role in this vital return of blood to the heart.

Diaphragmatic breathing stimulates the *peristalsis,* the wavelike-squeezing motion of the intestines which promotes digestion and the elimination of solid and semi-solid fecal wastes. Making a change from chest breathing to diaphragmatic breathing has helped thousands in correcting heartburn, gas, indigestion, chronic constipation, and liver problems, etc.

Often we seek to grow or change ourselves by adjusting the external aspects of our lives. We all too often forget that permanent or real change comes when our inner drives and motivations undergo transformation. – Errol Strider

43

Bragg Super Power Breathing Calms the Nervous System

The *solar plexus* is the *powerhouse* of the body. It's a network of nerves and ganglia (independent groups of nerve cells) which controls every important vital organ in the abdominal cavity and is located in the very center of the diaphragm. The more stimulation you give your diaphragm, the more circulation your solar plexus (often called the gut) receives. This increases the amount of nerve energy that is then available to your vital organs. The extremely important pneumogastric nerve (*pneuma* – lungs; *gastro* – stomach) passes through the diaphragm and also benefits from this diaphragmatic action.

Diaphragmatic breathing has a tranquilizing rhythm, stimulates your circulation and helps rejuvenate the body. B-complex vitamins also have a calming effect on the entire nervous system. Diaphragmatic breathing breaks up the paralyzing nerve tension so often observed in people with supersensitive or jangled nerves. For more details about the beneficial effects of deep breathing on the nerves, read our book *Build Powerful Nerve Force*. (See pages 174-175 for Bragg book information.)

Yoga teaches that deep, rhythmic breathing attunes one to the *rhythm of the universe* – in other words, one lives in rhythmic harmony with Mother Nature. *Prana*, the sanskrit word for *breath*, also means *absolute energy* or *vital cosmic energy*. According to the teachings of yoga, when we breathe correctly we store this energy in the solar plexus.

The Ayurvedic Health and Fitness Lifestyle

An ancient healing system developed in India thousands of years ago, Ayurveda (means science of life) is reemerging as an important model of health and fitness. In the ancient teachings of Ayurveda, a person's mind-body type is determined and specific diet, exercise and lifestyle routines are prescribed that are best for them, according to their mind and body type.

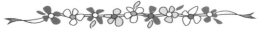

Just by paying attention to breathing, you can access a level of your relaxation and health that will benefit every area of your life. – Deepak Chopra, M.D.

44

Ancient Yoga Breathing Promotes Health

Essential to Ayurveda is the daily practice of yoga stretching and the importance of breathing correctly. Yoga breathing helps the mind and body become one. Learning to breathe correctly helps you remain calm in your daily living, during exercise and in stressful times.

Yoga breathing is nose breathing. For centuries, this has been known to slow the heart, lower blood pressure and relieve stress. Because it is a more efficient way to get oxygen into your body, it will enhance athletic performance. To practice it, start by doing some yoga stretches. Then walk with gradually increasing speed – breathing only through your nose – until you are jogging. When you can no longer nose-breathe easily, slow down until you can again breathe comfortably through your nose. Do this back and forth several times – jogging, walking, etc., always breathing through your nose. Finish with enjoyable yoga stretches. Practiced regularly, this calms you and gives you a greater oxygen capacity intake and increased energy, health and vitality.

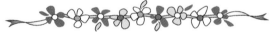

BAD NUTRITION – #1 Cause of Sickness

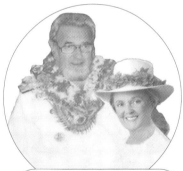

People don't die of infectious conditions as such, but of malnutrition that allows the germs to gain a foothold in sickly bodies. Bad nutrition is usually one of the main causes of noninfectious, degenerative or fatal conditions. When the

Dr. Koop & Patricia
Website: www.drkoop.com

healthy body has its full vitamin and mineral quota, including precious potassium, it's impossible for germs to get a foothold in its healthy bloodstream and tissues! We greatly admire our friend, the former U.S. Surgeon General Dr. C. Everett Koop who, in his famous 1988 landmark report on nutrition and health, stated this strong statement:

Diet-related diseases account for 68% of all United States deaths!

WHERE DO YOU STAND?

POSTURE CHART

	PERFECT	FAIR	POOR
HEAD			
SHOULDERS			
SPINE			
HIPS			
ANKLES			
NECK			
UPPER BACK			
TRUNK			
ABDOMEN			
LOWER BACK			

Your posture carries you through life from your head to your feet. This is your human vehicle and you are truly a miracle! Cherish, respect and always protect it by living The Bragg Healthy Lifestyle. – Patricia Bragg

Good posture helps prevent backaches and related problems.

Remember – Your posture can make or break your health!

46

Chapter 9

The Importance of Doctor Good Posture

Sit, Stand and Walk Tall for Health!

Humans – from head to feet – are built to stand, sit and walk erect. Now that we have reviewed the way your breathing apparatus operates, you can readily understand how correct posture is essential to correct breathing. When you slump, you squeeze your lungs and other organs into a cramped position that seriously limits the operation of your diaphragm. You become a shallow breather, able to use only the top portion of your lungs. When you sit bent over a desk, you rob your body of maximal oxygen intake, impair circulation, hamper the functions of your heart and vital organs and crowd your muscles and bones into unnatural positions. Then you wonder why you're so fatigued! You probably also cross your legs, which further blocks circulation, and prepares the way for broken capillaries, varicose veins, backaches, headaches and a host of other problems.

It is likely that you maintain the same poor posture when on your feet – standing or walking with your shoulders and head drooping or neck upthrust. You cannot improve matters by suddenly going to the opposite extreme: distorting your body and all of its components by an exaggerated reversal (i.e., thrusting your shoulders back and sucking in your stomach). You will improve and maintain good posture by strengthening your muscles with the daily practice of correct posture habits. *Start now – It works miracles!*

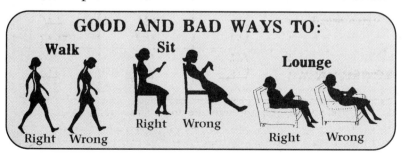

GOOD AND BAD WAYS TO:

Walk — Right — Wrong

Sit — Right — Wrong

Lounge — Right — Wrong

Learn by doing – Remember practice makes perfect.

Posture Can Make or Break Your Health!

Why should emphasis be placed upon such a simple thing as the pull of gravity? In your youth, your muscles held your skeleton in proper balance free from strain or discomfort. Perhaps now circumstances have caused your muscles to lose the battle with gravity. Maybe premature ageing, excess weight or an enforced rest has weakened your muscles just enough to cause your frame to be in an uncomfortable state of balance.

This sagging stretches the ligaments of your back and causes backaches. Ligaments that are stretched too far are painful. They are meant to serve only as check reins for the joints and cannot be forcibly stretched without pain. When the ligaments in your back are made uncomfortable by excessive stretching, it is natural for your muscles to try to oppose this gravitational pull. However, if your muscles are too weak to do their proper job, they will rapidly become exhausted and develop the misery of fatigue, making your back painful and uncomfortable.

PERFECT POSTURE AND ALIGNMENT

Check your own symptoms! Do you notice a deep aching and soreness along your spine due to stretched ligaments? Are your back and shoulder muscles achy and tired? Do you have a postural backache caused by weak muscles? If so, start now to strengthen your muscles with proper posture and exercise.

Your Health Friend is Doctor Posture

Look at yourself in the mirror! Do your **POSTURES** shoulders slump? Is your upper back round? Do you have a potbelly? Are you swaybacked? Can you see the reasons why your back has the right to ache? The bending, slumping, ligament-stretching force of gravity has finally taken charge. Even though you might be a sufferer of backaches due to poor muscles and bad posture, don't despair. With good exercise and good posture habits, plus living The Bragg Healthy Lifestyle you can regain your back and joint comfort!

WRONG   RIGHT

Backaches Afflict Over 31 Million Americans

It has been said that backache is the penalty people must pay for the privilege of standing and walking upright on two feet. Although some people erroneously believe our ancestors walked on all fours, it is an indisputable fact that we are definitely two-footed. Infants struggle instinctively to stand on their two feet and walk. They need not be taught! They attempt a bipedal mode even if left alone most of the time and never instructed. It's absolutely natural for human beings to stand and walk in this manner. This is especially interesting in light of the fact that no other animals spend all of their standing and walking hours on two feet, not even the primates that are most like us – chimpanzees and the great apes.

These animals use their hands and arms to help move them about. The world's strongest gorilla would be unable to follow a fragile human about, walking erect on his legs, for more than a short time. This is because we human beings are designed to walk upright and animals are not!

The spines of human beings have normal curves which enable the muscles to oppose gravity and hold the back erect. As long as the muscles are strong enough to maintain the balance and prevent sagging, the back is comfortable. When muscles are too weak to work, the back sags, ligaments are stretched and then the inevitable happens – a backache, that affects 31 million Americans.

Good posture is an important part of breathing. For correct posture, align your body with an imaginary vertical line from the top center of your head through the center of your pelvis to the floor between your feet. Do the posture exercise on page 52 often.

Establish this simple, incredibly beneficial habit: stand tall, walk tall and sit tall. When this healthy posture becomes a habit, the result is correct posture! Any sagging, prolapsed vital organs will slowly assume their normal positions and function better. Follow The Bragg Healthy Lifestyle daily and drink 8 glasses of distilled water and practice good posture.

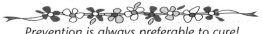

Prevention is always preferable to cure!

Learn to Stand, Sit and Walk Tall
For Body Strength and Super Health

To maintain and keep yourself in a healthy state involves many factors including healthy natural food, deep breathing, exercise, rest, sleep, control of emotions and mind, fasting and good posture. If you nourish and give your body loving care, good posture is natural. Conversely, when your body lacks any of these essentials, poor posture is usually the result. Once you have established poor habits, you will have to take definite and corrective measures! You will need to exercise regularly and practice good postural habits in order to restore your natural, healthy stature.

When you sit, your spine should be straight against the chair and both feet should be squarely on the floor or a foot stool. Your abdominal cavity should be well drawn in. Keep your shoulders back and hold your chest and head high, never forward. Your arms may be relaxed or you may lightly clasp your hands in your lap.

When you walk, imagine that your legs are attached to the middle of your chest. This will give you long, gliding, graceful steps. When you walk correctly with this swing and spring, you will naturally build energy. Habit either makes or breaks us. Good posture habits help make graceful, strong bodies. Remember . . .

As the twig is bent, so is the tree inclined.

When you sit, keep your torso up and relaxed. Sit squarely on your bottom (it's padded). Keep feet flat on the floor or with ankles lightly crossed. You can work for hours at your desk in this position without fatigue, but it's best to stop hourly for a good body stretch. Stand, stretch your spine up and do some shoulder rolls forward, then backwards. Then for more energy do some arm-wide swinging windmills. Also take frequent brisk walks, maintaining healthy posture with your arms swinging and breathing deeply in rhythm with your stride.

When sitting never cross your legs! Under the knees run two of the largest arteries, carrying nourishing blood to the muscles below the knees and to the nerves in the feet. You immediately cut down the blood flow to a trickle when you cross your legs. Don't cross your legs!

50

Don't Cross Your Legs – It's Unhealthy

When the muscles of the legs and knees are not nourished and don't have good circulation, then the extremities stagnate, which can lead to varicose veins or broken capillaries and other problems. Look at the ankles of people age 40 and over who have the habit of crossing their legs. Note the broken veins and capillaries. When the muscles and feet do not get their full supply of blood, the feet become weak and poor circulation sets in. Cold feet usually torment the leg-crosser.

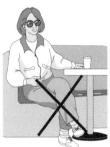

A well-known heart specialist was asked, "When do most people have a heart attack?" He answered, "At a time they are sitting quietly with one leg crossed over the other." When you sit, plant both feet squarely on the floor or a box if needed. Crossing your legs puts an unnecessary burden on your heart!

People who are habitual leg-crossers have more acid crystals stored in the feet than those who never cross their legs. Crossing the legs is one of the worst postural habits of man. It throws the hips, spine and head off balance and it's the most common cause of chronic backaches, headaches and varicose veins.

Poor posture can bring an unbearable pain across your upper back and fatigue in your drooping shoulders. It can also cause soreness that shoots from the back of your throbbing head to the base of your neck and downward to mingle with the stiffness in your lower back. Poor posture can cause weakness in your hips and loins, a numb feeling at your tail bone and often, a shooting pain down your legs. Bad posture can develop aches and pains all over the body. Be kind to your body and please don't cross your legs. You can break this habit.

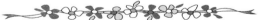

Poor posture inhibits the flow of oxygen throughout the body. With less oxygen taken in, every cell in the body then becomes undernourished and hungry for fresh oxygen. Of paramount importance is the circulation to the head area. Because of gravity, blood carrying oxygen naturally has to work harder to get up above the heart into the head. When poor posture interferes with circulation it also affects the skin, eyes, brain and hair. – Philip Smith, *Total Breathing*

Happiness is a rainbow in your heart – a real health sparkler! – Patricia Bragg

Bragg Posture Exercise Brings Miracles

Stand tall with feet nine inches apart. Tighten your butt and suck in stomach muscles. Lift up rib cage, stretch up spine, hold chest up, shoulders back and lift chin up slightly. Line up your spine – put finger on nose, plumb line straight to belly button, drop arms to sides and swing them to normalize your posture. Look in the mirror to see improvements. Do this posture exercise often; wonderful changes will occur! You are retraining and strengthening your muscles to stand straight for a healthier, fit body with more energy and youthfulness. Stand, walk and sit tall!

Practice good posture – do this exercise daily!

Which Posture Do You Have?

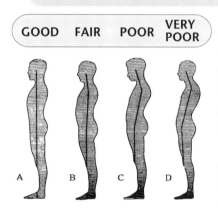

GOOD	FAIR	POOR	VERY POOR

A   B   C   D

How we stand and how we sit affects how we breathe. If the body is slumped over, the shoulders become rounded and the rib cage collapses, giving the lungs no room to expand. Notice the difference in your ability to breathe deeply when you are slumped over a desk and when you are sitting erectly, giving the lungs a chance for maximum expansion.

A) **GOOD:** Head, trunk, thigh in straight line; chest high and forward; abdomen flat; back curves normal.
B) **FAIR:** Head forward; abdomen prominent; exaggerated curve in upper back; slightly hollowed back.
C) **POOR:** Relaxed (fatigued) posture; head forward and down; abdomen relaxed; shoulder blades prominent; hollowed back.
D) **VERY POOR:** Head forward and down; exaggerated curve in upper back; abdomen relaxed; chest flat-sloping; hollowed back.

Wear Loose, Comfortable Clothing

Don't spoil your health with restrictive clothing such as tight belts, collars, undergarments, bras (see page 139) and even tight shoes for they can hamper breathing, blood circulation and the functioning of major organs. It can also throw your body and posture off balance. Today teenagers tend to wear clothes either too loose or too tight!

Cold Water Swimmers are Fit and Ageless

My father prides himself on being able to endure the coldest weather wearing only a small amount of clothing, and he has enjoyed swimming in all parts of the world, in all kinds of weather, (which I also enjoy). He is well known for his cold water swimming and is welcomed as a member at Polar Bear Clubs worldwide.

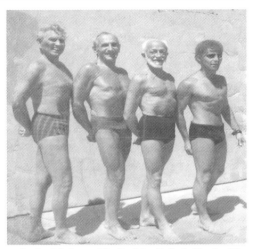

Dr. Paul C. Bragg 89, Dr. John H. Federkiewicz 77, David Cooper 70, Dr. David Carmos 27
Cold Water Swimmers at "L" Street Beach, Boston

On many occasions, Dad and the famous pioneer Dr. Robert Jackson had great sport breaking the ice and swimming with the amazing Boston Brownies of the famous "L" Street Bath House in Massachusetts. Here you'll find some of the finest ageless physical specimens in the world, including people in their 60's, 70's, 80's 90's even some over 100 years of age.

The same is true of the Polar Bears of Coney Island and at Montrose Beach in Chicago and those at the popular Bradford Beach in Milwaukee, Wisconsin. They are all fit, amazing and ageless. These healthy, hearty people who enjoy swimming in ice-cold water are all deep, full breathers. Many of them follow our Bragg System of Super Power Breathing. When you Super Power Breathe, you enjoy cold water swiming because both deep breathing and swimming are invigorating and energizing.

We certainly don't recommend that everyone jump into ice-cold water! Let's leave that to the people who have developed bodies with perfect thermostatic control. You can start slowly with alternating cold and warm showers. These swimmers are just examples of the power your body can develop when you are filled with oxygen at all times. There is no limit to your powers of resistance or your feeling of well-being when every cell in yur body is filled with precious life giving oxygen!

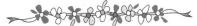

Studies show that athletes tend to have higher HDL (good cholesterol) levels.

Opera Singers, Ballet Dancers and Champion Athletes are Deep Breathers

Breath control, by deep diaphragmatic breathing, is vital for all professional singers. Without benefit of loudspeakers, the voices of the early great opera singers filled the auditoriums of the Metropolitan, La Scala and other famous opera houses throughout the world. What diaphragms they had! Look at the builds of these men and women. They have beautiful, perfect posture; superior development of the torso and tremendous lung capacity. Listen to the great recorded classic voices of Enrico Caruso and Mario Lanza, and those of other tenors who thrilled the world, such as Luciano Pavoratti, Placido Domingo and Jose Carreras. Hear their perfect voice control, from the softest pure note to the swell of a great crescendo. Study the lives of these extraordinary people and you will find that, regardless of their age, their attention to health and deep breathing filled them with energy and charm. Most of these deep breathers live remarkably long, productive, happy lives.

Secret of The Dancing Greats: Diaphragmatic Breathing

The same is true of all great dancers. Dad's friends, Ruth St. Dennis and Ted Shawn, thrilled audiences throughout their long lifetimes, from their teens into their 70s. Deep diaphragmatic breathing was the key to the tremendous energy and muscular control they brought to their spectacular dances. It was also the main key to their long, healthy, vibrant lives.

Deep diaphragmatic breathing is a basic component of the rigorous training of all the famous ballet companies. Many of the great dancers such as Fred Astaire, Gene Kelly, Arthur Murray and the rollicking Rockettes of New York's Radio City Music Hall were committed to The Bragg Healthy Lifestyle. In order to have super energy, dancers find it is important to live a healthy lifestyle. As a result, most live long lives, maintaining perpetual youthfulness. (P.S. *I've danced with Fred Astaire, Gene Kelly, Lawrence Welk & Arthur Murray – dancing helps keep you young!* – Patricia)

The beauty, strength, energy and endurance of North African dancers amazes me. Their secret is the excellent development of the diaphragm in breathing. Because their lungs draw in and expel large quantities of fresh air, these women have exquisite skin tone and flawless complexions, sparkling eyes and remarkably graceful and supple bodies.

Even if you aren't a singer or dancer, there is no reason why you shouldn't also enjoy good health and a long, happy, productive life. Without having to undergo the rigorous training of a professional performer, you can profit from their key secrets: deep diaphragmatic breathing, regular exercise, a healthy lifestyle and a natural diet.

Normalize Figure with Good Posture & Exercise

You can actually create a more fit body and a normal figure by using correct posture and breathing exercises and living The Bragg Healthy Lifestyle – begin now! All deep breathing exercises are body-building exercises. This is because oxygen is the invisible food, the life-giving miracle force of the body's 75 trillion cells and the vital compliment of the body's assimilation of dietary food. These exercises will help build up a person who is underweight and trim down a person who is overweight.

You can burn off fat by internal combustion. You can tone your body and keep it that way. Start now to normalize your figure into its naturally pleasing curves with correct deep breathing habits, along with brisk walking, regular exercise and healthy, wholesome food.

To be alive and thrill to the joy of living, you must learn to breathe correctly! Relearning correct breathing habits helps you to attain and maintain the healthy breathing practices you had as a baby. You must learn to breathe with every cell of your lungs. It is then and only then that you can raise your rate of physical vibration to its highest level for super energy.

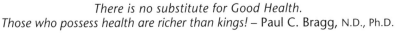

There is no substitute for Good Health.
Those who possess health are richer than kings! – Paul C. Bragg, N.D., Ph.D.

Good Posture – First Step to Healthy Living

Poor posture puts your heart, lungs and all of your *working machinery* into a viselike grip which impairs operations, circulation and efficiency. Keep saying to yourself, *"I must stretch up tall and lift up my chest and diaphragm."* Now, you will be exercising during all of your waking hours. Good posture brings inner strength and tone to your organs and muscles that no exercise can provide.

Correct posture is vital for health and longevity. Keep a straight line from the chin to the toes when standing. Don't slump in your chair when sitting. Keep the head, chest and diaphragm held high. This may tire you at first, but only because your unused muscles are being re-awakened and trained! Once you give strength and tone to the many muscles that control your posture (some also help hold your internal organs), you will find it's easy to maintain good posture. The health rewards are many and you will look and feel healthier and more youthful.

No One Can Breathe for You

You can build a new figure, a new You – inside and out – vibrant, healthy and tingling with the joy of life. Remember, You and You Alone have this great power to breathe deeply – You are Your Captain, it's all up to You!

This self-power to breathe deeply has no value unless it is used every day. You can build better blood circulation by daily doing The Bragg Super Power Breathing exercises and living The Bragg Healthy Lifestyle. You will soon become oxygen recharged and not feel fatigued at the least physical effort. Prove this to yourself – start today!

Breathing exercises bring sparkle to your eyes, a glow to your flesh and add vim and vigor to your step. You will be more mentally alert. Your reflexes will function better. You will feel fit and have a sense of well-being that is a far greater treasure than any material possession!

Oxygen is the most valuable of all nature's elements and you can have all you can breathe for free. You have only to learn how to fully utilize it with Bragg Super Power Breathing. By practicing long, slow breathing and taking longer, deeper breaths per minute you will enjoy greater health, more endurance, vitality, energy and a youthful life!

Chapter 10

Preparing for Bragg Super Power Breathing

Overcoming the Effects of Bad Breathing

The Bragg Breathing Exercises and Healthy Lifestyle work to tone and regulate your entire body to make it healthier. Most humans are victims of two bad habits: shallow breathing and incorrect posture. These habits must be overcome. Muscles must be strengthened, especially those of the diaphragm and the abdominal muscles. Unused lung air sacs must be opened and revitalized.

Perhaps you have already experienced a *stitch in the side* when you have had to run to catch a bus or plane, or while doing some unaccustomed exercise. Actually this can be a good sign, if you will profit by it. It is good to exercise to the point of getting that *stitch*. What it really means is that you have discovered a large area of unused lung cells, which have remained closed most of your life, since childhood. Now your lungs are opening to receive the fresh air you are pumping in through your efforts to breathe more deeply. The diaphragms of older people can become semi-paralyzed from non-use, but exercise and Bragg Deep Breathing can change that!

As lung cells suffer disuse they begin to stick together and collapse in upon themselves. The sharp pain is due to the air forcing these cells apart. Continue to breathe deeply, even after you have caught the bus, plane or stopped your exercise, run, etc. The distress soon passes and your unused lung cells will soon become reactivated. You will then have made an important step forward in Bragg Super Power Breathing and achieving greater super vitality and health.

If you experience that *stitch* during the preparatory exercises which we are going to outline, you will now understand what it is caused by and not be alarmed. Just keep on deep breathing for more super energy!

Breathing is the greatest pleasure in life. – Papini

57

Practice Bragg Posture Exercises Every Day

Correct posture allows the chest to expand so that the lungs can be filled with air. The lungs inflate with air like millions of tiny balloons. Suction is created below by the action of the diaphragm and above by the auxiliary muscles of the chest and abdomen. This suction fills your lungs with air. <u>The lungs themselves are passive and cannot breathe independently. The lungs wait patiently to be refilled with air. So now make it a habit to breathe deeply</u> to help keep your lungs and body healthy.

Remember, the lungs are attached to the rib cage walls by pleural membranes. If the sternum, or breastbone, is carried high and the bony rib cage expanded, the lungs are held up in position so they can be filled with air. The uplifted diaphragm, in turn, tends to draw into position the sagging or prolapsed organs of the abdomen.

As with deep breathing, most young children exhibit good posture naturally, only to lose both as they mature. To make matters worse, most occupations today (from assembly line to desk jobs) have a tendency to pull us down from an erect, good posture position. The result is that many people carry themselves like a collapsed accordion, shoulders sagging, chest deflated, which puts their heart, organs and breathing apparatus in a tight viselike grip.

1 A special exercise is needed to counteract this unhealthy and energy-sapping poor posture. Stand with your feet 10 inches apart. Now stretch your hands high overhead, at the same time rising high on your toes. See how high you can lift up your chest while drawing in the abdominal muscles. Stretch up and up, as if trying to touch the ceiling. *Repeat this posture exercise 10 times.* Do not try to do any special breathing. Just breathe naturally, or what is natural for you at the time.

This exercise is designed to strengthen the muscles which control the erect posture of the body. Stretching is one of the greatest tools for building health. It is the universal exercise of the animal kingdom. Wild animals are beautiful examples of instinctual natural living. Also, house pets (cats, dogs, birds, etc.) all stretch daily. *Whenever you've been sitting for a while, do this stretching exercise.*

Stomach Muscles Need These Exercises

Most people allow their stomach muscles to be lazy, flabby and unhealthy. A good time to strengthen, tone and control these muscles (your natural girdle of muscles) is to practice this every morning before you get out of bed. Remember your waistline is your lifeline.

2 Lying on your back – fix your eyes and attention on your stomach. Now start moving your stomach muscles upwards, then force them downwards. Wiggle your insides, in one direction, then another, then from side to side, letting your hands help at first. When you discover you can control your muscles in one movement, then practice the other movements.

Thinking about and using these stomach muscles is just the beginning. The goal of these exercises is the ability to control the abdominal muscles in the same way you do those of the legs and arms. Your stomach muscles must do your bidding if you want to develop a useful diaphragm. After you have obtained some control over your stomach muscles while lying on your back in bed, *begin doing the same movements while standing upright.* You can accomplish much more in this upright position.

3 Standing upright, with hands hanging relaxed at sides, draw in and up the stomach muscles until it looks like a deep valley, as though everything inside was moving up in the chest cavity. Then push your muscles out until you are surprised of your protruding belly. Now suck the muscles in, then push out. Now wiggle them up and down, and last pull in, tighten, firm and stretch up your midsection and spine. Repeat several times.

When you acquire this control over the abdomen and surrounding muscles, you will discover many benefits. A huge reward is that you will also establish a more normal bowel rhythm. Usually upon arising and within an hour after each meal, there should be a bowel movement. (See exercise on page 69.)

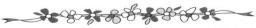

Your waistline is your healthline, dateline, youthline and lifeline! – Patricia Bragg

He who can't find time for exercise will have time for illness. – Lord Derby

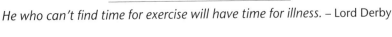

59

Diaphragm Exercise

When exercising your abdominal muscles, you will also be exercising your diaphragm, especially in the upward and downward pushing movements. Here is a special exercise for your diaphragm: *locate your diaphragm* by placing one hand at your waistline, then with the other hand hold the palm upward in front of your mouth. Now blow imaginary dust from the palm. Where you feel a strong muscular contraction when blowing, that's the location of your **diaphragm, the most important muscle you use in Bragg Super Power Breathing.**

4 Walk around your room on your bare tiptoes, with your hands stretching up, reaching high over your head. Raise your diaphragm as high as your strength will allow you to lift it, still breathing deeply. Feel it stretch the chest and stomach muscles as you breathe deeply. Now bend over, drop head below your heart, arms towards floor, then circle your arms in front of chest, compressing out every bit of old toxic, carbon dioxide-laden air. Do this often, as it's a super lung cleanser and health builder.

It's a great habit to suck the oxygen-bearing fresh air deeply and slowly into your lungs. If you feel a little dizzy with the sudden oxygen stimulation, stop for a moment, then continue. *Begin by doing this diaphragm stretch – deep breathing exercise 5 times, gradually increasing to 10.* When you are able to do this exercise with ease, you are ready to start your Bragg Super Power Breathing Program (page 67).

Improper breathing is a common cause of ill health. Changing your breathing patterns can affect you emotionally and physically. – DrWeil.com

Apple Cider Vinegar Zaps Sore Throat & Laryngitis – *Organic, raw ACV is a dangerous enemy to all kinds of germs that attack the throat and mouth! To fight the germs and keep the throat healthy, an ACV gargle mixture works miracles (1 tsp. to ½ glass of water). Gargle 3 mouthfuls of mixture each hour, then spit it out. Don't swallow the gargled mixture, because ACV acts like a sponge, drawing out the throat mucus, mouth germs and toxins.*

– Bragg Apple Cider Vinegar Book

The beginnings of all things are small. – Cicero

Singing – Breathing Exercise

What is more elemental to singing than the breathing in and out of pure air into your hard-working lungs? Projecting sound and sustaining a note is the hallmark of strong breathing muscles just as a lean, firm body is the sign of healthy, fit living. With singing, just as in breathing, the diaphragm and abdomen take lead roles and this exercise will help you master their use.

While standing up straight, feet 10 inches apart, place your left and right hand fingers on bottom ribs with thumbs gently probing below bottom rib. Now slowly draw in a full, deep diaphragmatic breath while feeling 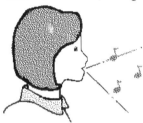 your abdominal movements with all fingers. Hold your breath for 5 seconds, now slowly exhale . . . but don't just "breathe out", instead, you should "sing out" the air. So, as you slowly let your breath out, softly sing a sustained note, as in "aa-hhh" or "oo-hhh". Note the abdominal movements with your fingers again. Repeat exercise 3 to 5 times. This helps you extend your control over the flow of sound and breath and helps you master your breathing machinery.

Candle – Breathing Exercise

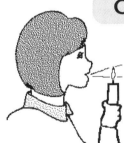 In this version of the singing exercise, instead of holding your sides you hold a candle in front of your mouth. Again, slowly sing out your breath as evenly as possible – and thus exercise mastery of your breathing by controlling the candle flame.

Arm Pumping – Breathing Exercise

Stretching up spine, stand tall, legs relaxed with feet 10 inches apart. Drop arms down at sides. Now gradually pump arms up and down bird-style, breathing in through your mouth until your arms are up above your head. Grasp hands, stretch up, hold breath for 5 seconds. Now slowly breathe out as you bend down, relaxed, dropping arms and head below your heart. Repeat twice.

61

Wise Thoughts for Wise Healthy Living

We are a product of our thoughts – and so is our health! While doctors and medicine have their place, <u>self-healing is the most powerful medicine of all</u>. Accepting the present and placing trust in a higher power frees your energy to focus on improving your life! See problems as challenges of growth, not as a punishment or judgement! <u>Focus on happiness, forgiveness, hope and peace of mind, as well as physical change to ease any problems and situations</u>.

Our Creator would never have made such lovely days, and given us the deep hearts to enjoy them, unless we were meant to be immortal. – Nathaniel Hawthorne

---

Change and growth take place when a person has risked himself and dares to become involved with experimenting with his own life. – Herbert Otto

---

A strong body makes a strong mind!
– Thomas Jefferson, *3rd U.S. President 1801–1809*

Every part is disposed to unite with the whole that it may thereby escape its own incompleteness. – Leonardo DaVinci

---

The body and the mind are so closely connected that not even a single word or thought can come into existence without being reflected in the personality and health of the individual. – John Prentiss

---

Studies show repeatedly that exercise – particularly impact exercises like brisk walking, tennis, square dancing, cycling, aerobics and weight lifting – help you maintain a healthier body and build stronger bones!

Exercise helps you lose and control weight in two ways. First, by elevating your metabolism you burn more calories. Second, by building muscle – which requires more energy to maintain – you use even more calories. Exercise promotes better elimination and circulation, which help body cleansing!

The breath and movement of Chinese medicine's Tai Chi; the breathing and body postures of yoga; and the ecstatic dances of native people around the world reflect the universal benefit of movement and deep, slow breathing. – Nini Beegan, *International Breathing Institute*

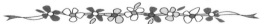

Exercise is good for your health, but like everything else, it can be overdone. Too much exercise hampers the immune system. Couch potatoes need to exercise 30 minutes every day, but those who run, do high-impact aerobics or lift weights need to take time off for the body to recharge and rest. A day of rest refuels your energy and motivation. Studies show that athletes who take rest days, like twice a week, actually improved their performance over those who trained every day. – Shape Magazine www.shape.com

Chapter 11

What is Bragg Super Power Breathing?

Basic Scientific Natural Laws

Bragg Super Power Breathing is based upon simple, natural laws. The more oxygen you get into the body, the more carbon dioxide poison you will eliminate from the body. When oxygen replaces carbon dioxide, there will be greater purification of the blood, cells and organs of the body for better health and a longer life.

Thousands upon thousands of lives have been saved with oxygen therapy. It is a well established scientific fact that, when all known conventional methods of healing fail, oxygen is used to save lives.

So, let's reason this out together. If pure oxygen can save the lives of humans who are on the brink of death, is it not logical that inhaling more oxygen deeply can prolong our lives? Or that it will free us from toxins that bring pain and distress to our physical bodies and, above all, give us a greater enjoyment of life?

Oxygen is the only stimulant upon which you can safely rely as a depression chaser and body builder. Bragg Super Power Breathing's main purpose is to get more life-giving oxygen into all parts of your body for health.

Bragg Super Power Breathing Exercises should not be confused with physical exercises. While this kind of breathing does produce more energy and physical and nerve strength, it has nothing to do with mere muscular development. However, it is almost impossible to have ample oxygen freely circulating in the body without beneficial effects occurring throughout. Extra benefits will be healthier muscle tone, more firmness of the skin and improved posture. Oxygen is a miracle normalizer!

Man's precious breath is the gift of life from God.
With the care and nurturing of this life gift, all health and wisdom is ours.

The basic principle of Bragg Super Power Breathing is to fill the lungs to capacity with oxygen, then hold breath in, leaning forward, drop your head below your heart. This uses the force of gravity to infuse the head's cavities with oxygenated blood, which energizes the brain and helps maintain and create new brain cells (see page 14).

Breathing Exercises Stimulate Pituitary Gland

Stimulation of the body's master gland, the pituitary, is one of the greatest benefits of Super Power Breathing Exercises. *The pituitary gland is located at the base of the brain and is the master of every human act and unconscious function occurring within the heart and abdominal cavity.* It determines a person's height and the length of their bones and the muscle and pulse strength, mental activity, and even the lifespan.

The pituitary is the master gland of life and controls the functions of all the other body glands. The more oxygenated blood you give the pituitary gland, the greater the output of all the valuable hormones of the body. The better the glands function, the more the entire body will rejuvenate itself to stay healthier and more youthful!

This is why the following exercises are called Super Power Breathing Exercises. Although each one is directed toward a specific part of the body, all employ the same basic, super oxygen principle. They all also stimulate the master pituitary gland and brain area with oxygen.

Enjoy Early Morning Breathing Exercises

Upon awakening in the morning it's ideal to first do some slow body stretching exercises. Then super-charge your day with a peak supply of oxygen energy by doing 10 to 15 minutes of Super Power Breathing Exercises. After your exercises enjoy a glass of our delicious Bragg Apple Cider Vinegar Drink (*1 to 2 tsps ACV mixed with 1–2 tsps raw honey (optional) in glass distilled water, recipe page 116*). For more info read *Apple Cider Vinegar –The Miracle Health System* and *Water – The Shocking Truth That Can Save Your Life!* (See back pages for Bragg booklist.)

Nature cannot be hastened. The bloom of a flower opens in its own proper time. – Paul Bruton

The early morning hours are especially important for doing these breathing exercises, especially if you are a city dweller, because the air is less polluted at this time of day. These exercises will start your day with a store of super energy that will carry you through whatever challenges may arise. You will become more confident, optimistic, stronger and healthier.

Think of this health-building period with pleasant anticipation. It's a time to build your vitality, energy, strength and all the good things that come to a healthy body. Go into it with dedicated self-responsibility and enthusiasm. Your faithful efforts will return super results!

Fresh Air and Warmth are Necessary

Sleep in a well-ventilated (airy) room on a firm mattress (memory toppers are nice). Use natural cotton percale or flannel sheets, also these and silk are preferred for nighttime wear, or wear nothing. Don't use electric blankets or heating pads, because they can disturb your body's natural currents according to scientists and even be harmful to your health. If you must, only use to prewarm, then unplug. A hot water bottle is safer.

Be sure there's ample fresh air circulating in your room. If not, do these exercises before an open window. We want you to get full benefit of these stimulation exercises and to enjoy every minute of it. If it's too cool when you get out of bed, put on something that is loose and warm. We often wear sweatshirts and sweatpants.

As you start doing your exercises you will soon feel a wonderful glow of circulation coming over your entire body as you become warmer. When you feel warm enough, peel off your sweat clothes and get right down to your bare skin. Give yourself an external as well as an internal air bath. Let your 96 million pores breathe in the breath of life, too. Remember that you also breathe through your skin! It's an important organ of respiration – Your skin is often called your *third lung*.

Love makes the world go 'round, and it's everlasting when it's given with caring, loving advice that will improve and enrich your life! This is why my father and I love sharing with you the health wisdoms which can be with you on your life's long happy journey. Our Bragg books on health, longevity and fitness go around the world spreading health and love! – Patricia Bragg

Air Baths are Health Builders

The pores of your body will welcome the contact with fresh air. They are going to be wrapped up in clothes all day and probably at night also, unless you sleep in the nude. Daily air baths (babies also) do wonders for the skin. No creams can give you *"skin you love to touch"* like fresh air can! A daily private (nude) air bath also greatly enhances your skin's primary function as the main thermostatic regulator (control) of your body's temperature. This practice helps condition the skin to adjust to hot and cold weather more easily. It's a faithful thermostat when you treat it well. But if you keep your body heavily clothed and overheated all the time, your skin becomes like a hothouse plant, unable to withstand drastic temperature changes. When you allow your entire body to breathe freely in the nude, your body's thermostat learns to readjust itself so that it works perfectly for you in hot and cold weather! (Also, try this powerful combination twice weekly: air bath and lite skin brushing on page 158.)

Breathe Through the Mouth and Nose

Let us make it clear that to breathe most effectively one should use both the mouth and nose to breathe normally. Our Creator has equipped your nose with hair miracle filters to strain out dust and pollens. It also has temperature regulating chambers (sinuses) to warm or cool the air before it enters the lungs, as well as moist mucus which traps particles missed by the hairs and expels them through the nose or mouth. The human body is also equipped with a larger, secondary air entrance, the mouth for use when a greater amount of oxygen is needed: during strenuous sports and exercise such as swimming, running, bicycling, tennis, aerobics, etc.

Since the purpose of Bragg Super Power Breathing is to fill the lungs with as much oxygen as possible, we use both the nose and mouth to breathe in and out. Do this exercise often – fill your lungs by breathing deeply in through the nose; pucker lips into a small opening; now exhale slowly and strongly with a hissing sound.

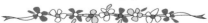

Now I see the secret of making the best persons, it is to grow in the open air, and eat simple and natural and sleep with Mother Earth. – Walt Whitman

Chapter 12

Bragg Super Power Breathing Exercises

Exercise 1 – The Cleansing Breath

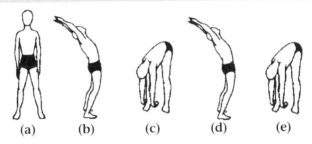

(a)   (b)   (c)   (d)   (e)

This is your basic Super Power Breathing Exercise. All Super Power Breathing Exercises begin this way. Stand erect, feet about 15 to 18 inches apart, hands and arms relaxed at your sides (figure a). Raise your hands overhead (figure b). Now bend forward as far as possible – keeping your knees slightly bent and relaxed – exhaling at the same time through your mouth. Compress your chest and push upward with your diaphragm and abdominal muscles to expel all the stale air from your lungs (figure c).

Now slowly inhale through your nose and mouth, pushing downward with your diaphragm and expanding your chest at its front and sides. Continue to draw in air to the full capacity of your lungs as you return to a standing position, while bringing your arms upward in a half-circle to the overhead position (figure d).

To complete the Cleansing Breath Exercise: As your hands reach the overhead position, then tighten your diaphragm and hold your breath for four or five seconds (mentally counting, *one thousand one, one thousand two,* etc.) while pulling your abdominal muscles back as if to pin your stomach to your backbone. Then exhale completely while bending forward, as in figure c & e. Now inhale as you return up as figure b and repeat exercise. Do this Cleansing Breath Exercise 5 times.

67

Exercise 2 – The Super Power Brain Breath

Start by exhaling and inhaling as in Exercise 1. When your hands reach the overhead position, hold your breath (hold nose closed if necessary) and bend forward from the waist, knees bent, dropping your head below your heart, downward as far as possible. Continue to hold your breath to the count of 10 (mentally counting, *One thousand one, one thousand two,* etc.). This exercise allows the richly oxygenated blood to suffuse the pituitary gland on its way to reaching, refreshing and recharging every part of your brain for sharper thinking (work, school, etc.). This power breathing also cleanses the skull cavities (sinuses, ears, nose, eyes and mouth).

While holding your breath, return to a standing position. Then bend forward, exhaling vigorously through the mouth. Slowly inhale as you return to starting position. Do this exercise 5 times at the beginning, gradually increasing to 10 repetitions.

NOTE: In these exercises, you may not be able to hold your breath for the full count at first. If you begin to feel dizzy, exhale and return to the standing position, dropping your arms to your sides and relax for a few minutes before continuing the exercise. You will gradually build your oxygen tolerance to the full count.

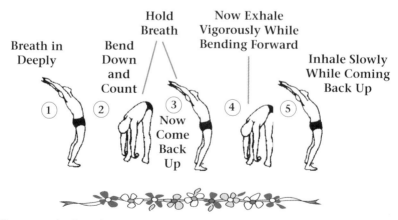

Breath in Deeply — Bend Down and Count — Hold Breath — Now Exhale Vigorously While Bending Forward — Inhale Slowly While Coming Back Up — Now Come Back Up

Viruses and microviruses (as flu, colds, HIV, arterial plaque and cancer cells) thrive best in low oxygen environments. They are anaerobic. That means increase oxygen level (deep breathing) around viruses, etc. and they die. – Ed McCabe

Man is fully responsible for his nature and his choices. – Jean Paul Sartre

Exercise 3 – The Super-Kidney Breath

Locate your kidneys on the lower back, just below the end of your rib cage near the waistline. Get the *feel* of them by placing your palms over this area, fingers and thumbs pointed downward. Use this position during the breath-holding part.

Exhale and inhale as at the beginning of Exercise 1. As your hands reach the overhead position, tighten your diaphragm and pin your stomach to your backbone with your abdominal muscles, while holding your breath. Then firmly place your palms, with light pressure, over kidneys (on back below waist) relax knees and bend backward for a silent count of 10 (*One thousand one, two thousand two,* etc.).

Still holding your breath, return to standing position. Then bend forward while exhaling vigorously through the mouth. (Use same precautions as in Exercise 2.) Slowly inhale as you return to the starting position. Do this exercise 5 times at the start, gradually increasing to 10.

Exercise 4 – For Easier Flowing Bowels

Do this exercise in the bathroom soon after rising each morning, and several times within an hour after eating. If you make this a habit, you will soon find you will have a bowel movement within an hour after eating.

Exhale and inhale as beginning Exercise 1. Now, holding breath, clasp hands in front and slowly lower yourself into relaxed squatting position while still holding your breath. Then strain for bowel movement for several seconds. Return to standing position and now by exhaling and inhaling as in previous exercises.

Note: Squatting is a natural way to have bowel movements. Children squat naturally. It opens up anal area more directly. Putting feet up on a wastebasket or footstool when on the toilet gives the same effect. Also stretch arms above head so the transverse colon will empty easier.

Eliminate the "Dribbles" Exercise

To keep bladder and sphincter muscles tightened and toned, urinate – stop – urinate – stop, 6 times, twice daily when voiding, especially after the age of 40. This simple exercise works wonders for men and women.

Health and intellect are two blessings of life. – Monostikoi

Exercise 5 – Filling the Lungs

This exercise is designed to get oxygen into the little-used air sacs at the bottom (apex) of the lungs, down near your waistline. Exhale and inhale as at the start of Exercise 1. But instead of returning the arms to the overhead position, relax them at your sides and bring your feet together, toes and heels touching. While holding your breath, bend to the right and reach toward the floor with the fingers of your right hand, at the same time bringing the left hand up to touch under the left armpit. Hold this position for a silent count of 10. Return to starting position and exhale and inhale as before. Now repeat the breath-holding position on left side. Reach toward floor with left hand while placing right hand under right armpit for count of 10. Repeat this exercise 5 to 10 times, alternating sides.

Exercise 6 – The Super Power Liver Cleansing Breath!

Exhale and inhale as at the beginning of Exercise 1. Now bring feet together and clasp your fingers overhead, palms upward. Keep legs stiff from the hips down. Now holding a full breath, bend slowly to right side, then the left side, with as much stretch as possible. Now after doing left and right side stretches, return

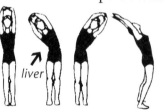

liver

to starting position, but with feet apart. Next exhale with the usual forward bend, forcing all the old air out and then breathe in as you come up. Do 5 sets, gradually increasing to 10 repetitions of this liver cleansing exercise that promotes cleansing and circulation.

Always do what is right – despite any public opinions.

The health of the people is really the foundation upon which all their happiness and all their powers as a state depend. – Benjamin Disraeli

There is no substitute for Good Health.
Those who possess it are richer than kings! – Paul C. Bragg N.D., Ph.D.

It's never too late to get into shape, but it does take daily perseverance.
– Dr. Thomas K. Cureton – Physical Fitness Pioneer, University of Illinois

Exercise 7 – Heart Strengthener

The purpose of this exercise is to expand the aorta, the main trunk of the arterial system which carries the blood from the heart after it has been oxygenated by Super Power Breathing. This exercise stimulates the circulation of blood in the heart, as well as the entire body, cardiovascular system, etc. It also helps recharge and increase the power of the respiratory system. This exercise also helps give relief to those who suffer from the feelings of suffocation and apprehension caused by asthma, angina pectoris, etc. (See Healthy Heart Habits page 138. Live a healthy lifestyle, plus drink 8 glasses of distilled water daily.)

This exercise starts with exhaling and inhaling as in the beginning of Exercise 1 (page 67), except that the arms are held forward at shoulder height (not overhead). When you return to the standing position, hold your breath – clasp your nose tightly with thumb and index finger so that no air escapes. Then pretend you are blowing your nose. You should feel some air pressure in your ears.

Now, with knees bent, bend over from the waist and gently bring your head down below your heart and midriff. Continue to hold your breath for a silent count of 10.

Return to the starting position and exhale and inhale in the usual Bragg Super Power Breathing manner (page 67). Repeat this exercise 5 times, gradually increasing to 10 repetitions.

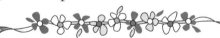

Coronary heart disease is due to a lack of oxygen received by the heart.
– Dr. Dean Ornish, _Author of Stress, Diet and Your Heart (www.amazon.com)_

_Nothing transforms anyone as much as
changing from a negative to a positive attitude!_

Breathing only in the upper chest avoids the strong creative energies of the abdomen and sexual organs. Breathing only in the abdomen avoids the powerfully creative energies of the heart and throat. – Michael G. White

---

If you are honest with yourself, you will quickly discover that most of the things we truly love to do in our leisure time are not only simple, but also free and surprisingly healthy. So, instead of rushing out to see the latest film or show, why not watch the sunset? Take a walk in nature alone or with a loved one! Read the Bible, a favorite book or listen to your favorite music!

Faithfulness Counts Towards Super Health

Every person who is interested in Super Health should take time each morning to do these Super Power Breathing Exercises. Take your present physical condition into consideration when you start on this program. Go slowly at first. Large parts of your lungs have probably been dormant for some time. It will take time to gradually open up these areas. Daily exercises will bring miracle results.

Make these exercises a daily habit, as much a part of your life as dressing, brushing your teeth and eating. The wonderful results obtained from faithfully following these breathing exercises and lifestyle will repay you abundantly with more health, energy, peace and longevity!

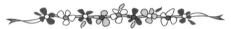

A wicked messenger falls into mischief;
but a faithful ambassador is health. – Proverbs 13:17

Accuse not nature, she hath done her part; now do thine!
– John Milton, *Paradise Lost*

Nourish the mind like you would your body.
The body and mind cannot survive on junk food.

CREATIVE MEDICINE

It is no over-simplification to say that our health comes from the soil. No matter how many physicians and health professionals we train, and how much curative or preventative medicine they may practice, we cannot attain optimum health until our attention is focused on preventative medicine, and thereby learn to keep and even improve our health. To build and maintain healthy soil is the real fundamental service. Creative medicine must be founded on growing healthy organic foods. Thus alone can we create real health for our people – only through creating a sound, healthy and prosperous organic-minded agriculture. – Dr. Jonathan Foreman, *The Land*

MONDAY TO JOY-DAY

There are days when you feel buried in the blues. You get up feeling depressed and pessimistic. You look worried. The world just isn't spinning in your direction. Yesterday you had it on a string, but today it has you beneath its weight. What to do? We should realize that we are destined to have these days from time to time. They are as natural as rain. If we were always happy we'd not appreciate our joys. If we didn't have hard knocks, we wouldn't appreciate the pleasant times so much. Maybe it takes Monday morning blues to make a week well-balanced. – Dr. J. DeWitt Fox, *Health Culture*

Chapter 13

Learning Breath Control

You Enjoy More Health and Happiness

Your lungs can hold at least 6 pints of air. If you keep your lungs filled to capacity you will feel better, have more energy, suffer less fatigue, sleep better, wake up refreshed and be a healthier, happier person. With practice you can learn to control your breathing, taking only 6 - 8 long, full breaths per minute for a healthier and more energized productive life. Prove it – start now!

Evening and Bedtime Routines

At the end of your work day and after activities, make it a habit to refresh yourself with some stretching, a few Super Power Breaths and diaphragm exercises. This will help cleanse the impurities from your body that have accumulated throughout the day. You will then be ready for dinner and a more relaxed, healthier evening.

Just before bedtime, remove your clothes, relax and stretch every inch of your body. Then slowly and deeply inhale and exhale. Now you're ready for bed, put on comfortable nightwear, for sound sleep is a miracle recharger and a time for your evening meal to be digested and it's life-giving nutrients assimilated!

Deep, Full Breathing Helps Relieve Pain

Civilized human beings with their unhealthy, self-destructive eating and living habits tend to accumulate latent poisons in their bodies. This means that the body stockpiles toxic poisons in different areas when they could not be disposed of through the body's regular avenues of elimination. These poisons are stored in veins, arteries, joints, organs, tissues, skin, etc. When they accumulate and press on nerves and tissues there is pain. You may think this pain is new but it's usually a *flare-up* of old stored-up body toxins (except in cases of injury).

The quality of breath should be deep, graceful, easy and efficient. – Kenneth Cohen

73

Heed Warning Pains – Eliminate Cause

Don't take pills to ease warning pains – find the cause and eliminate it! Live The Bragg Healthy Lifestyle! <u>Use oxygen to help burn the poisons out of your body</u>! There's absolutely no better way of flushing toxic poisons out of the body than by the powerful action of oxygen. Ample power breathing, 8 glasses of pure distilled water daily, and fasting, are the greatest natural purifiers on earth! For instance, <u>you may have a pain in your right foot which is quite common, since the force of gravity will often cause toxins to settle in the legs and feet</u>. Painful gout is a perfect example of this tendency.

Now let's get the toxins out of that right foot! Exercise as follows: lie flat on back, take a long, deep breath and hold it. While holding your breath, raise left leg, bend at knee, and with both hands pull and press your leg against your chest as you exert the full downward force of your diaphragm at the same time. You will feel oxygenated blood flowing unrestrictedly down into your right foot. Now slowly exhale. (Also never sit with legs crossed.)

This same technique may be applied to any part of the body. For example, for a headache, take a full breath (exhaling and inhaling as in Exercise 1, page 67). Holding the breath, relax your shoulders and bend your head downward below your heart. This allows a free flow of oxygenated blood to the cavities of the head and brain. <u>Headaches are also helped by fasting and the herb</u> *feverfew*.

Aches and pains from fatigue are nearly always due to stagnant venous blood filled with toxic carbon dioxide and congestion in various parts of the body. Swollen ankles, for instance, generally occur due to an accumulation of venous blood and water bloating. Exercise and Super Power Breathing will help to activate circulation and return blood to the heart. From the heart it will be pumped to the lungs, where the carbon dioxide will be exchanged for body purifying oxygen.

"Relieved of the work of digesting foods, fasting permits the body to rid itself of toxins (headaches, etc.) while facilitating healing. Fasting regularly gives your organs a rest and helps reverse the ageing process for a longer and healthier life. Bragg books were my conversion to the healthy way."
– James Balch, M.D., Co-Author *Prescription for Nutritional Healing*

Exercise Relieves Varicose Veins & Leg Swelling

If you sit or stand for a long time and your ankles become swollen, lie flat on your back, raise your legs and stretch your feet toward the ceiling and breathe deeply. It also helps to circulate any stagnant pooled blood (varicose veins) by using your hands to gently press downwards from ankles to hips. You will feel the blood flowing from your feet and ankles toward your heart. If you are in a place where you can't do this, breathe deeply in and out while you alternately rise up on your toes, then down and up on your heels. The deep breathing and muscular action will stimulate circulation, and help relieve the venous blood congestion and provide relief for aching legs and feet. These are good exercises upon awakening and before bedtime.

Power Breathing & Brisk Walking Exercise

Of all the many forms of exercise, brisk walking is the one that brings most of the body into action. It is the *king of exercise* and when the rhythm of your deep breathing and the rhythm of your stride are in harmony, you feel more vibrant and alive! Practice these breathing exercises faithfully to gain perfect control of your breathing and to become a tireless walker. As the oxygen-filled blood courses through your body, your legs will carry you along buoyantly. Walk tall with your head held high, back straight, chest up, tummy in, arms swinging easily from your shoulders; legs moving as smoothly as though they were attached to the middle of your torso.

Enjoy your walk with a free spirit and a light heart. Start at your own pace to fit the movement – fast, medium, or slow. Watch with interest the things and people you pass, or let your walking be an accompaniment to your ideas and thoughts. As you breathe and walk rhythmically, awareness of your body will diminish. You will become more at peace and in tune with Mother Earth and God.

You can truly *walk your worries away!* As the blood courses through your arteries and veins, cleansing and nourishing your entire body, you become filled with a sense of well-being. This cleanses your mind of its troubles and nourishes it with positive, healthy, happy thoughts.

Brisk Walking is the King of Exercise

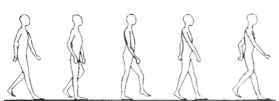

Walking Posture

Always prepare a new foot base before leaving the old one.

As we stride along on our walks we say, "Health, Strength, Youth, Vitality, Peace, Love, Joy, Eternity!" With walking you discover the beauty of God and Mother Nature as it awakens, softens and enriches your soul and life! Walk briskly at least one to three miles every day and more when you have time. Don't make excuses! Make your daily walk a fixed routine no matter what kind of weather. In stormy weather, walk inside your home, on your porch or driveway, in the mall, etc. When traveling, use hotel hallways, stairs or even the treadmill or exercise equipment in the hotel's gym. Walking can be done anytime, anywhere. Start today!

Dad and I always prefer outdoor fresh air walking, but walking indoors is far better than no walking at all. When traveling the world on our Bragg Health Crusade tours, we often take a light jog or a brisk evening walk through the corridors of our hotel or up and down the hotel stairs. Our favorite places for brisk walks are beaches, hills and the open decks of cruise ships.

Miracle – Walking Builds New Blood Vessels

American Health reported that Dr. Gary Giangola, a vascular surgeon at New York University Medical Center, prescribed walking instead of bypass surgery for one of his patient's atherosclerosis. It was so pervasive it had severely restricted the blood flow to the legs and was causing extreme pain and numbness in his patient's feet. Dr. Giangola told his patient that if he walked one mile every day (even if he had to stop every two blocks to recover), he would build new blood vessels (collaterals) which would bypass his closed arteries. He enjoyed his recovery!

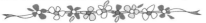

Recent studies revealed that fat stored in the body's "spare tire" around the waist increases risk for diabetes, heart disease and other serious health problems! Studies shocking fact: the bigger the waistline, the shorter the lifespan!

Super Power Breathing Makes Exercise Fun

One year later the patient was able to enjoy walking several miles daily. Walking and living The Bragg Healthy Lifestyle is fun and promotes miracles! The results of surgery are often risky, life-threatening and temporary, unless they are combined with permanent lifestyle changes that include a healthy diet and exercise, etc.

Whether your preferred exercise is walking, hiking, jogging, biking, aerobics, swimming, golfing, dancing, calisthenics, tennis, weightlifting or any other aerobic activity, you will reap greater benefits from it when you establish the correct habits of the Bragg Super Power Breathing. Plus, you will have super energy to exercise more often and you will have fun enjoying it more!

Super Power Breathing Calms the Nerves

The greatest tranquilizer for jangled nerves is deep, slow, diaphragmatic breathing. Today's tensions and pressures put additional strain on our nervous systems. The condition is aggravated by poor posture habits and shallow breathing. Your Bragg Super Power Breathing Program will help you correct both of these unhealthy habits . . . while having a calming, healthy effect on your nervous system and entire body!

During your workday, take at least a minute out of every hour to pause and s-t-r-e-t-c-h from your toes to the top of your head while doing deep, diaphragmatic breathing! Do back and forward shoulder rolls as well! The small amount of time invested in this program will pay dividends in productivity over the course of your day, because you will be able to do your work faster and with greater efficiency. This is especially important for those restricted to desks, but it's helpful in any kind of work, even manual labor. By oxygenating and relaxing your nerves, you will no longer be distracted or upset by petty annoyances at work or those minor irritations with fellow workers, the boss or your friends or family.

Everything has its wonder, even darkness and silence. – Helen Keller

There is a positive side and a negative side and at every moment you decide. – Sister Corita

B-Complex and Magnesium
Improves Breathing and Soothes Nerves

When an emotional upset occurs, which inevitably befalls each of us occasionally, go off by yourself and take slow, long, relaxed breaths. Soon you'll find your nerves quieting down and more logical thinking will replace emotionalism. You will become master of the situation and better able to calmly resolve your problem. (Magnesium, B12, B-Complex or their injections help breathing, calm the nerves and improves brain function. St. John's Wort also helps.) Read our book *Build Powerful Nerve Force* for info on improving your nerve health.

Deep Breathing Helps Respiratory Ailments

Letters and case stories give testimony to the blessed relief that Bragg Super Power Breathing has brought to thousands suffering from breathing problems such as sinusitis, bronchitis, asthma and emphysema. These suffocating diseases, characterized by chronic mucus inflammation and obstruction of the air passages, have become more prevalent today as our air becomes more polluted. (Take precaution, use air purifiers and humidifiers for home, office and your car. *See page 95*) In fact, colds, flu and chronic sinus inflammation are the most common illnesses seen by doctors today. Backaches are second.

Many people suffering from respiratory problems fail to understand that these are often naturally occurring body responses to an unhealthy toxic lifestyle (wrong foods, milk, toxic air, etc.). They hope nasal sprays will relieve their breathing problems. Many don't follow directions and abuse the sprays, often becoming addicted with disastrous consequences. Nasal spray abuse can cause a secondary illness, *rhinitis medicamentosus,* when the nose becomes inflamed by the medicine drug itself.

To help relieve these symptoms safely and naturally, do a simple Apple Cider Vinegar Nasal (sniff) Wash. Add ½ tsp. Bragg ACV to cup of warm distilled water. Cup in hand, sniff up left nostril, roll head back, then side to side, lean over bowl, blow out mucus. Then repeat with other nostril, do 3 times. Do 2-3 daily until mucus conditions subside. Also enjoy Bragg ACV Health Drink 3 times daily (recipe page 116).

78

Some Common Respiratory Ailments

Respiratory diseases are becoming more common all over the world, particularly in industrialized countries like the United States. Air pollution, cigarette smoking and congested, overcrowded living conditions are some of the main problems. The average human inhales 3,000 gallons of air daily. Unfortunately millions breathe contaminated, toxic, sick air in their home, offices, cities, planes, etc.

• **Bronchitis:** Bronchial inflammation. *Prevention:* Healthy lifestyle, no damp climates, no smoking, no polluted cities. *Treatment:* Diet, rest, 8 glasses daily distilled water, breathing exercises, use steam inhaler, hot herbal chest packs. (Read page 81.)

• **Asthma**: Bronchial swelling. *Prevention:* Healthy lifestyle, see list of helpful preventions and treatments on pages 38-40.

• **Hyperventilation**: Breathing is short, fast panting. *Treatment:* Healthy lifestyle. Breathing into paper bag (3 minutes) helps to restore carbon dioxide/oxygen levels in the lungs.

• **Emphysema**: Lungs loose elasticity and normal functioning. *Prevention:* Healthy lifestyle, breathing exercises, no smoking.

• **Lung Edema**: Accumulation of fluid buildup in the lungs. *Prevention:* No cold, damp, smoggy climates, no smoking. Coughing should not be suppressed. Breathing exercises. Eat lightly, do fasting. *Treatment:* Heimlich Maneuver, administer oxygen, rest and as a last resort, have specialist tap lungs.

America's National "Sleep Debt"

The National Sleep Foundation poll taken recently discovered that a whopping 67% of American adults have a sleeping problem and that over one-third (37%), are so sleepy during the daytime that their daily activities are interfered with. Over the past 100 years, we've reduced our average sleep time by 20% and, over the last 25 years, added an additional month to our annual work/ commute time. Our national "sleep debt" is rising and while our society has changed, our physical bodies and needs have not. We are paying dearly for such "progress"! Visit their interesting website: www.sleepfoundation.org

Help me Lord, to know the magic of rest, relaxation and the restoring power of sleep.

The average person spends about 23 years of a 75 year average lifespan asleep.

Getting Enough Sleep Lately?

The odds are you are not getting sufficient sleep. American adults presently average 7 hours nightly. While everyone's sleep needs vary, most scientific research indicates that we require 8 hours of sleep nightly. Few are lucky enough to enjoy 5 to 6 hours of sound sleep and still perform well at work. To just get "caught up," a full ten hours of rest, plus naps are frequently called for!

First make a clear choice about how you wish to spend the thirty to forty-five minutes that precede your actual going to bed. Avoid a rush to "get things ready for tomorrow" or to catch up on tasks not completed during the day. This is a time to read, relax and rest your body and mind. Try a aroma herbal bath or a (Bragg olive oil) self-massage while showering, hour before bed – it's so relaxing. Enjoy a warm soothing Bragg Apple Cider Vinegar drink with cinnamon and honey (recipe on page 116) or a Lemon Balm or Sleepytime herbal tea before bedtime.

Lemon Balm, whose scientific name is *melissa officianalis,* is a soothing plant with both nervine and antiseptic, relaxing natural qualities. It's a member of the peppermint and spearmint family and is grown worldwide. When flowering it has a lemon fragrance – a perfume delight.

Healthful Tips for Sound, Recharging Sleep

- Avoid stimulants such as caffeine (found in coffee, tea, soft drinks, chocolate, sugar) and nicotine (found in cigarettes and other tobacco products).

- Don't drink alcohol to "help" you sleep, it's unhealthy!

- Have herbal teas – anise, lemon balm, sleepytime, chamomile, or try melatonin, tryptophan (5HTP), valerian, calcium and magnesium supplements; they work miracles.

- Exercise regularly, but try to be finished with your workout no sooner than 2 hours prior to bedtime.

- Establish a regular and relaxing bedtime routine; for example, enjoy a warm aromatherapy bath or shower.

- Associate your bed with recharging sleep – don't sit on it to work or watch TV. *Try memory 2" foam topper on mattress.*

- If you suffer from insomnia, don't nap during the day. Remember, you earn better sleep by daytime activity.

Relief for Stuffy Noses & the Snorer in the House

Finally here's a drug-free solution for the snorer, etc. This breakthrough is simply a nasal strip, an adhesive band-aid-like device that helps keep open the nose's nasal passages and allows easier airflow during sleep. There available in pharmacies, sizes small to large. Cost about 25¢ a night. This allows those with stuffy noses, the snorer and those nearby to have a restful sleep. Also there's a simple laser surgery that helps if needed.

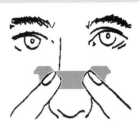

A nasal strip in this position on the nose helps snorers and those around them get a good peaceful night's sleep.

Help for Bronchitis and Asthma

When people suffer from bronchitis and asthma, the mucus membranes of their bronchial tubes have become inflamed. The brain (human computer) triggers the release of more mucus in an attempt to soothe and heal the irritation. Unless this mucus is decongested and expelled, it clogs these vital air passages. With asthma, even the tiny bronchioles (the smallest branches of bronchial tubes in air sacs) become swollen. Victims feel like they're suffocating, and in severe cases, they do! Try 4 drops of lobelia tincture on tongue when needed – page 39. Prolonged chronic bronchitis and asthma can often progress into lung distructing emphysema. This causes the air sacs to become so distended with trapped stale air that they lose their elasticity, and they can slowly suffocate. <u>Super Power Breathing can't restore destroyed tissue, but it can help salvage and revitalize the rest of the lungs</u>! The life-giving inflow of oxygen acts as a natural decongestant and gradually cleans out the bronchioles and bronchial tubes. This helps remove toxic carbon dioxide and other waste from the air sacs and lung tissues. This cleansing and opening-up of the lungs helps revitalize every possible cell with more oxygen and nutrients!

After years of asthma, within a month I could breathe almost normally for the first time in my life. It was a miracle! I thank Paul Bragg and the Bragg Fasting & Breathing Books – Paul Wenner, Creator of Gardenburger – Author, Garden Cuisine

Actress Cloris Leachman is an ardent health follower who sparkles with health. She hates smoking, coffee, alcohol, sugar and meat. One of her solutions to health problems is to fast. "Fasting is a miracle cure, it cured my asthma."

> *Important: it's absolutely essential that you eliminate all cow's milk and its products from your diet, as these produce mucus and sickness!*
> See info on web: www.notmilk.com & antidairycoalition.com

Respiratory ailment victims have gained permanent relief by following <u>The Bragg Healthy Lifestyle and eliminating all milk products, yogurt, cheese, butter, ice cream, etc., along with fasting for a 24 hour period weekly and eating a healthy vegetarian live foods diet.</u> Do your breathing exercises, gradually increasing walks and other exercises. <u>Take vitamin C, bioflavonoids and CoQ10; they promote lung tissue healing and help reduce any bronchial wall swelling.</u> Read page 31 for more supplements to take and read these Bragg Books: *The Miracle of Fasting, The Bragg Healthy Lifestyle, Apple Cider Vinegar,* and *Water – The Shocking Truth.*

Help For Asthma Attacks

Contrary to common belief, asthma attacks are not caused by an inability to breathe (inhale), but rather by an inability to exhale the dirty stale air collected in the lungs. Try the following technique for relief of an asthma attack. Someone close to you needs to learn this Heimlich Maneuver, because it's difficult to do it for yourself.

Stand behind the person having the attack, wrap your arms around the torso in a hug, and then, using both hands, lift the entire tummy and diaphragm upward, as if you were trying to push it up under ribs and breastbone. (This Heimlich Maneuver is similar for a choking person, read pages 130-131.) When they can breathe easily again, have them get down on their hands and knees, straddle them and repeat process. This technique helps the diaphragm return to its normal, healthy position easily. If the attack is severe and this technique doesn't work, be sure to follow your regular medical program.

Reduce Asthma Trouble Triggers

It's important to identify and reduce your asthma triggers. The most common include tobacco and smoke; chemical sprays, gas fumes, perfumes, car exhaust; pollen; mold; animal dander; sudden changes in temperature or weather; certain medications such as aspirin; and food additives including sulfites and MSG.

90% of our metabolic oxygen comes from breathing. 10% comes from food.
– Dr. Gabriel Cousins, Author; "Conscious Eating" available Amazon.com

Controlled Deep Breathing For Super Oxygen

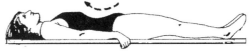

1 Do this exercise before getting up in the morning and repeat often during your day. It's also relaxing just before sleep. Count to yourself as you gently exhale and slowly inhale (vary breathing through mouth and nose). When you become more adept then increase the count.

It's challenging to have breathing contests with family and friends to see who can take the deepest, slowest, longest breaths. This exercise will strengthen your lungs, chest and all of the muscles around your midwaist. It also improves your lung capacity and super breathing power as it gives you a firmer, trimmer waistline. This will help you learn to breathe in and out with control, varying breathing through the mouth and nose. When on walks pay attention to how long it takes to inhale and exhale. Ideally exhaling should be longer.

Diaphragmatic Panting Breathing Exercise: Super Oxygenator For Super Healthy Living

2 Raise your arms so that your ribs are separated. Rather than breathe as you normally would, pant while breathing. Pant until your diaphragm is tired. Your exhale panting should take about twice as long as your inhale panting. For example, if your inhale lasts for a count of 6, try to make your exhale last to 12. Do this exercise daily, especially before retiring. This helps re-oxygenate your entire body and removes toxins from your system so you can enjoy a more restful and rechargi

Poor posture inhibits the flow of oxygen throughout the body. With less oxygen taken in, every cell in the body then becomes undernourished and hungry for fresh oxygen. Correct posture is a contributor to the overall health of the body. The spine is the major conductor of nerve messages through the body. Its health is critical to the proper functioning of all sensory and regulatory organs.
– Total Breathing by Philip Smith (www.amazon.com)

Bragg Books can be your faithful health guides, by your side night and day.

One-Breath Meditation Works Miracles

3 ATP (adenosine triphosphate) is a naturally occurring by-product of breathing that regulates physical action, thought and feeling. Dips in ATP levels can cause fatigue, aches and pains. The one-breath meditation exercise reverses falling levels of ATP.

A *Sit in a comfortable chair and straighten your spine, keeping shoulders back and relaxed.*

B *Now inhale slowly and deeply, and clear your mind completely. Relax your shoulders and back. Imagine yourself in your secret garden, deeply drawing in peace and vitality from the oxygen rich air.*

C *Hold your breath for a moment, then exhale slowly and fully, releasing all tension from your muscles and body.*

Use this one minute refresher at home, work and throughout the day as needed to refresh, restore and recharge your body, mind and soul.

Breathing Exercises During Pregnancy and Childbirth Benefits Mother and Baby

In natural childbirth classes (waterbirth, birthing chair, etc.) parents are taught certain breathing techniques, as Lamaze or Bradley, to help make childbirth easier and more comfortable. Visit www.lamazevideo.com & www.bradleybirth.com. Mothers who practice Bragg Super Breathing throughout their pregnancies have stronger muscles. This enhances their ability to make use of other breathing techniques and helps make the birthing process easier. This ensures that the mother and baby will have a healthier, happier, birthing experience.

The primary benefits for the mother are a shortened recovery time and the ability to fully participate in the joyful process of her child's birth. For the baby, the primary benefit comes from the well-oxygenated blood the mother had been providing for the 9 months she carried the child in her womb. This oxygen helps prevent birth defects and helps ensure that the baby is born healthier and ready for a long, normal, healthy life!

Learn about Waterbirth, see websites: waterbirth.org & ecstaticbirth.com

Breathing is the greatest pleasure in life. – Papini

Chapter 14

Breathing Exercises To Enjoy For More Energy

The Bragg Super Power Breathing exercises are powerful for super health. Here are ways to add more variety for your enjoyment. Make some or all of these exercises a part of your daily routine to give you more super vitality, health, creativity and fitness in your life.

Posture Breathing Exercise

The following activity is designed to correct bad posture habits, which are among the greatest impediments to proper breathing. Practice this activity several times a day at the job and at home. It will bring relief to your tired shoulders, spine and eyes, making you more alert and energized.

While sitting relaxed in a chair, let your chin rest on your upper chest as you slowly lean forward, exhaling. With eyes closed continue leaning until hands and elbows rest comfortably on your upper legs. After slowly exhaling in this position, sit upright quickly while sniffing in a full breath of fresh air through the nose. As you do this let your eyes open wide and then hold your full breath for 10 seconds (if necessary, first begin with holding for 5 second counts).

Take special note of how the sudden inhalation works to force your posture to healthy alignment as you sit up straight. After holding the inhaled breath, slowly release air through the mouth. Then close your eyes, lean forward and then repeat the exercise two more times.

Nerve Force contains much of its power in the breath. – Yoga Teachings

---

As a single footstep will not make a path on the earth, so a single thought will not make a pathway in the mind. To make a deep physical path, we walk again and again. To make a deep mental path, we must think over and over the kind of thoughts we wish to dominate our lives. – Henry D. Thoreau

Super Power Breathing for Fresh, New Air

Because the majority of people don't use their full lungs' capacity, the following exercise is designed to get new air into the forgotten, unused regions of the lungs. Practice moderately at first, but with greater frequency as your lungs become healthier and stronger.

Comfortably sit or stand and now inhale slowly through the nose a complete, deep diaphragmatic breath. As you do this let your head be comfortably lifted backwards until it has come to rest as far back as it can without strain. After holding this position and your breath for 3 to 5 seconds, slowly exhale through closed teeth as your head moves forward to the starting position. As you exhale (there should be a hissing noise as the air is forced between the teeth) concentrate on expelling all of the old air out of your lungs. Repeat this exercise several times. It's particularly suitable to pre-aerobic warm-ups because it prepares the lungs for super oxygenation.

Rejuvenation Breathing Exercise

When areas of the lungs have remained unused, the pathways can become narrowed or even closed. This breathing exercise helps rejuvenate the lungs by opening up the passageways to the lungs' neglected areas. Do this activity moderately and gently at first. But as your lungs become healthier and stronger, increase the frequency and force of your exertion.

While standing, take in a deep, full diaphragmatic breath and lift your chin up slightly. Once you have taken in the full breath, hold it in and stand still. Then raise your bent arms chest high and with closed fists gently pound your upper chest area (still holding your breath) in gorilla style. Also pound your rib areas and the lower lung region. Do this for as long as you can comfortably hold your breath. As you exhale, knees relaxed, bend head down below heart and exhale as much old air as possible from your lungs. Repeat this exercise several times.

To desire to be healthy is part of being healthy. – Seneca

With a full breath swelling your lungs, this gentle pounding (patting) exercise opens up those passageways that haven't carried air for a long time. The more passages you have available to move air through your lungs and into your blood, the more energy and vitality and better health and fitness you will experience.

Exercise to Increase Lungs' Air Space

This breathing exercise helps you make use of your lungs' maximum breathing capacity in a comfortable and gentle manner. Practice several times a day for more energy and fitness on the job and at home.

While standing, knees relaxed, bend over and exhale completely all the old stale air. You can help your lungs expel (push out) the air by pulling in your belly muscles, forcing your stomach inwards towards your spine. Now stand straight, slowly inhale, filling your lungs to full capacity and hold your breath for 20 seconds (if 20 seconds is not possible, set a challenging, non-painful goal). As you count, slowly stretch your arms up over your head. This will stretch your lungs, maximizing their air space. When you have completed your breath holding pattern, relax and bend down and exhale air slowly. Do this 2 or 3 more times and increase as desired.

Exercise for A Flexible, Youthful Rib Cage

As with the preceding exercise, this maximizes the body's spatial capacity for breathing. The previous exercise works on increasing the lungs' air holding capacity. This exercise works on the space your rib cage can make available for your lungs to expand.

While standing, exhale completely with arms at your sides. Slowly inhale, filling your lungs to capacity and hold your breath for 20 seconds. As you count place your palms on your hips with your thumbs forward and your pinkie fingers touching each other at your lower spine.

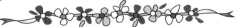

We must always change, renew, rejuvenate ourselves; otherwise, we harden.
– Johann W. Goethe

Now pull elbows backward far as possible while holding your breath. Then exhale slowly moving arms down to sides. Repeat 2 or 3 times. This exercise helps keep the rib area flexible, to maximize air lung space.

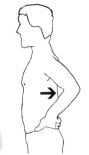

Exercise To Maximize Chest Area

This exercise will also help you maximize the available chest and rib cage area for your lungs to expand and take in more air. Practice several times daily along with the other air capacity increasing exercises.

Starting position – stand with arms at sides, inhale deeply through the nose, then while holding your breath for 5 seconds, extend arms forward, now clasp hands together and stretch hands up, high above your head, exhaling quickly and fully through your mouth. Naturally your upper chest will move upward with this stretch. Now return to starting position and repeat 2 or 3 times.

Breathing Exercise for Lower Lungs

The lungs' lower regions are the most distant from your windpipe, and the most dependent on the breathing activity of the diaphragm. As a result, the lungs' lower regions are the most likely areas to suffer disuse. This exercise is designed to bring air to these underused areas of the lungs.

While lying on the floor on an exercise/foam pad concentrate on your lower lungs. Put tip of index finger just below your belly button and consider this spot the center of your lower lungs. Slowly inhale through the nose a full and total breath, concentrating on filling the lung area beneath your finger first. With practice you will soon find that you can easily target your breathing in this way. As you inhale fill your lower lungs first (beneath finger), moving to your familiar upper lungs last.

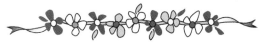

Exercise, exercise your powers; what is difficult will finally become routine.
– George C. Lichtenberg

After a few days of practice your skill level in this exercise will noticeably increase and you will find it easy to aim your breathing to different regions of your lungs. Once you have this ability, practice this exercise while standing or lying down, at home or at work. You will find that it is both soothing and invigorating, suitable both for before sleep and for energy when tired.

Deep, Slow Breathing Promotes Better Sleep

Millions worldwide suffer from insomnia – bad sleep and bad sleeping habits. Preparing sensibly for a night's rest (ventilated room, firm mattress with memory 2" foam topper) is one of the easiest ways to improve your ability to sleep well. The following deep breathing exercise relaxes the body and reduces mental stress to prepare for a peaceful, recharging sleep so vital to your health.

Lie in bed on your back with hands at your sides, palms down. Close your eyes and quiet your mind as you slowly inhale through your nose attempting to fill your lower lungs first. As you inhale, raise your arms in a slow arching, circling motion up over your head. Aim to complete your inhalation just as your 2 thumbs touch each other, with arms resting behind your head on bed. Hold this breath for 10 to 15 seconds. Exhale slowly through your mouth as you reverse your arm circling motion, bringing arms back to starting position at sides. Repeat exercise several times or until relaxed and drowsy.

Stop Procrastinating – Start Exercising Daily

When it comes to these exercises - and in fact all exercises and all habits of sane and healthy living - what is truly important is the DOING. "Knowing" and "wanting" are important too - but "doing" is what it is all about. Don't play counter-productive games with yourself. The moment you begin asking yourself, "Do I have time to do this right now," is the very moment to stop asking and start doing! The moment you begin to think, "I don't have the energy right now," is the very moment to stop thinking negatively and start doing. Be positive, start now, please no more procrastinating!

Exercise, deep breathing, healthy foods, with some fasting helps maintain a healthier physical balance in our daily living for a longer, happier life.

Start the 10 Minute Trick – It Works Miracles

The successful student of The Bragg Healthy Lifestyle, and anyone who has successfully made healthy exercise part of their daily routine, will tell you the same thing: The moment of beginning is the most difficult. The in-between moment after you decide you want to become healthier and before you begin to act on that decision is the hardest moment. The moment before you put that one leg in front of the other on the first step of your brisk walk is the most difficult moment of the exercise.

The people who tell the success stories of exercise recommend "tricking yourself" into exercising at first. Play the "10 minute trick". Before you start (the hardest moment), tell yourself, "I'll only exercise for 10 minutes and then I'll stop. That will be easy and I'll be done soon." Once you've done this, you're on the path to healthy fitness - and it will be fun! Once this most difficult moment is over (the beginning) you'll find when the 10 minute mark comes around that you are enjoying yourself too much to quit so soon.

Fast Help for Panicky, Stressful Moments

Stress and fear tightens the entire body, especially the breathing muscles. Learn to relax and loosen the tightened muscles and panic and tensions will melt away.

These simple-to-do exercises will bring fast relief:

- Concentrate breathing in deeply and slowly, then blow out slowly all the stress and tension.
- Wait! Don't breathe for a few seconds. While breath is out, force stomach muscles in and out 4 times.
- Slow shoulder rolls to ears – then roll back, down and around, then reverse rolls.

Do 5 times and you will be more relaxed and peaceful.

For a nervous stomach, do this finger acupressure:

Firmly press your skin between thumb and forefinger. This helps for car and plane sickness and a nervous stomach. Life is a journey of choices, relax, be healthy, happy, peaceful, enjoy your healthy lifestyle and count all your blessings!

Chapter 15

Oxygen Depletion And Air Pollution

The Urgent Problems of Air Pollution

These days it doesn't matter where in the world you live or where you go, you can no longer absolutely escape exposure to the poisons that we humans have mindlessly dumped into our air, water and land. In pristine Minnesota, your water might be dangerously contaminated from upstream paper pulp mills. On beautiful New Guinea beaches, you might have to step around hazardous garbage carried great distances by ocean tides. Toxic waste by-products from oil production are everywhere in Middle East deserts.

What these places all have in common from India to Mexico, from California to London, is air pollution. This is the greatest and most pervasive scourge of modern man. Some areas are far worse than others. My recent travels bring London and Los Angeles to mind. The smoke contamination of the early industrial revolution compared to today's more deadly toxic chemical revolution is almost out of control. When air pollution toxins can actually be seen, then it's called *smog.*

What Is Smog?

Smog is a general term that refers to the various kinds of visible air pollution. The word *smog* – a combination of the words *smoke* and *fog* – was first invented in Glasgow, Scotland in the early 1900s. It described the thick, bad air that plagued and continues to plague their city. This smog killed over 1,000 people in 1909! Smog today is more complex than simply smoke mixed with fog. Many of these toxic pollutants are invisible to the eye. Reread pages 35-37. Visit www.epa.gov-www.arb.ca.gov

Pure, clean air is the invisible staff of life!
Smog is the invisible staff of death.

Smog is a Deadly Health Hazard

Today we fortunately have national and local agencies whose job is to prevent such past horrible smog disasters. These agencies constantly monitor air pollutant levels and atmospheric conditions. Based on their findings, stronger guidelines and legislation will likely be implemented to protect our health, but problems do persist. Environmental Protection Agency (EPA) notes that a larger number of Americans are living in areas that don't meet air quality standards. Over 64 urban areas don't meet federal standards of air quality – standards which many say are not safe enough to keep our air healthy! (www.epa.gov)

When industrial pollutants and car exhaust react with sunlight, dangerous chemical reactions occur. The most dangerous of these produces ground-level ozone O_3. Ozone, the Earth's protective layer high above our planet, guards plant and animal life from the sun's damaging ultraviolet radiation. Yet at ground-level, where we eat, breathe and live, ozone combined with pollutants is responsible for smog's trademark "haze". This has a smothering toxic effect on the city dweller on smoggy days causing choking, coughing and eye-burning.

In many ways the problem of smog is worse now than 50 years ago. Hopefully we will never have air pollution disasters on the scale of some in the past. No one wants to live through suffering like that of the disastrous London smog attack of December 1952. A thermal inversion settled a fog on this great city on the Thames, trapping the pollutants spewed from its heavy industries and thousands of chimneys. Before the crisis abated, more than 4,000 people were dead and countless had fallen ill. Hospitals were inundated with patients suffering from cyanosis, a condition in which a person actually turns blue for want of oxygen!

Recently, the EPA approved new, more protective air quality standards. According to EPA estimates, these new standards will prevent "15,000 premature deaths yearly, 350,000 cases of aggravated asthma and 1 million cases of decreased lung function in children." Because of these new standards, many cities and urban areas will monitor air and become more alert to air pollution problems.

Dangerous Ground-level Ozone Smog

"Ground-level" ozone, a key component of smog, damages human lungs, animals, crops, even buildings and paint. Some areas are considered "serious" by the EPA (Environmental Protection Agency) who plan to clean up the environment in America. (www.epa.gov)

According to the EPA, cars and trucks contribute more than 50% of the locally-generated air pollution. The remainder comes from solvent evaporation, surface cleaning and coating, petroleum production and marketing, other mobile sources (boats, trains, planes), combustion engines and other miscellaneous sources.

The health effects of ozone focus on the respiratory tract: asthma, bronchitis and other respiratory disorders are worsened by high ozone concentrations. High ozone concentrations are especially harmful to children, the elderly, those with respiratory illnesses and people who exercise outdoors, walking, jogging, biking, etc. in smog.

It's best to become politically aware of all situations that affect your health in the region where you live. Vote for the laws and strong regulations that protect your health rights, especially to breathe clean, non-toxic air!

Clean Air Act Benefits and Costs

According to EPA study back in 1998, The Clean Air Act cost Americans about half-a-trillion dollars and provided a benefit of $21.5 trillion. Benefits were looked at for a number of factors, including improved public health and avoided food crop damage. If the Clean Air Act had not been enacted by 1990, 205,000 Americans would have died prematurely and millions more would have suffered from respiratory illnesses ranging from mild to severe!

Throughout the Clean Air Act, questions have been raised as to whether the health benefits of air pollution control justify the costs incurred by industry and taxpayers. The broader question is simple: How do the overall health, welfare, ecological and economic benefits of the *life-saving* Clean Air Act compare to these high cost programs? The saving of human and animal health and our food crops is reason enough to continue with programs to clean up the air, to protect lives and crops!

Let's Clean Up Our Air – For Our Health

Paving over land increases overall temperatures – and ozone forms more quickly at higher temperatures. More than one-half of commuting trips and 3 out of 4 shopping trips are less than 5 miles in length – perfect for cycling. For example: if Santa Barbara County could replace just 3% of its car and light truck trips with bike trips, they could reduce emissions of smog-forming pollutants in this California county by 9 tons monthly.

We Need the Protection of the Clean Air Act!

The results indicate that the benefits of the Clean Air Act and associated control programs substantially exceeded costs. A second important implication of this study is that a large proportion of the cost benefits of the Clean Air Act reducing comes in two major smog pollutants: lead and particulate matter. Not only monetarily, but from a health standpoint as well, the Clean Air Act is vitally needed and important!

Rank	Metropolitan Area
\multicolumn{2}{c}{**15 Worst Cities for Smog – Air Pollution***}
1	Los Angeles - Long Beach - Riverside, CA.
2	Fresno - Madera, CA.
3	Bakersfield, CA.
4	Pittsburgh - New Castle, PA.
5	Eugene - Springfield, OR.
6	Salt Lake City - Ogden - Clearfield, UT
7	Sacramento - Arden - Arcade - Truckee, CA.
8	Cleveland - Akron - Elyria, OH.
9	Visalia - Porterville, CA.
10	Birmingham - Hoover - Cullman, AL.
11	Detroit - Warren - Flint, MI.
12	Washington, DC - Baltimore, MD.
13	Louisville - Elizabethtown - Scottsburg, KY - IN
14	Chicago - Naperville, IL.
15	Provo - Orem, UT.

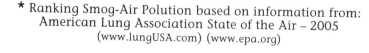

* Ranking Smog-Air Polution based on information from: American Lung Association State of the Air – 2005 (www.lungUSA.com) (www.epa.org)

Healthful Solutions to Air Pollution

How can you supply your lungs, your blood and your whole body with clean healthy oxygen in this modern era of air pollution? Oxygen, our invisible staff of life, is the great purifier and detoxifier, the body's basic life force. First you must protect and strengthen your nose and sinuses, your lungs' first line of defense. <u>Don't drink or eat any dairy products, for they increase mucus production and cause airway passages to swell</u>. These conditions hinder your nose's ability to filter the air you breathe, which is needed to protect your lungs and health. Take care of your nose, sinuses and health! Also develop powerful lungs that can withstand the challenges of polluted air when in it.

Action 1 Do your Super Power Breathing Exercises in the early a.m. when air is cleaner and less contaminated.

Action 2 If you live in a smoggy area (*moving is best when possible*), it's important to install the best Hepa air filters available – particularly in rooms you sleep, exercise and work in, office, etc; even have one in your car. Learn how to clean the filters and replace the pads so that they are always clean, washed and able to cleanse and purify the air. Buy filter pads in long strips and cut them to fit.

Action 3 Fortify yourself internally with a multiple vitamin-mineral supplement, ample vitamin C and especially vitamin E (natural d-alpha mixed tocopherols), the body's oxygen protector. One of the vital functions of vitamin E is to regulate the use of oxygen by the body's cells. This helps assure that your life-giving oxygen is properly utilized for essential energy and that a reserve is retained in the red corpuscles for use when extra effort is needed. According to documented medical research, <u>vitamin E helps increase the energy potential of all the oxygen you breathe by an amazing 25% to 50%!</u>

Cleanse the Air in Your Home, Office & Car!

Many people are unaware that exposure to indoor pollutants at home and work is often greater than levels outdoors, causing serious health problems. Having an air purifier helps eliminate bacteria, viruses, mold, and other indoor pollutants. Read Consumer Report 5/05 & visit these webs for more info on clean home air: www.oreck.com, www.iqair.com

Now I see the secret of making the best persons, it is to grow in the open air, and eat simple and natural and sleep with Mother Earth. – Walt Whitman

<u>*Premature ageing is a highly toxic condition caused by shallow breathing, nutritional deficiencies, toxic air, negative thinking and an unhealthy lifestyle!*</u>

Vitamin E Antioxidant-Rich Healthy Foods Are Important for Your Health & Longevity

A partial list of foods that contain the following amounts of precious, healthy Vitamin E. This list was compiled from *The Bridges Food and Beverage Analysis.*

Food	Quantity	Vitamin E IU's
Apples	1 medium	0.74
Bananas	1 medium	0.40
Barley	½ cup	4.20
Beans, Navy	½ cup	3.60
Butter (salt-free)	2 tablespoons	0.80
Carrots	1 cup	0.45
Celery, Green	½ cup	2.60
Corn, Dried for Popcorn	1 cup	20.00
Cornmeal, Yellow	1 cup	3.40
Corn Oil	2 tablespoons	29.00
Eggs, Fertile	2	2.00
Endive, Escarole	½ cup	2.00
Flour, Whole Grain	1 cup	54.00
Grapefruit	½	0.52
Kale	½ cup	8.00
Lettuce	6 leaves	0.50
Oatmeal	½ cup	2.00
Olive Oil (virgin)	½ cup	5.00
Onions, Raw	2 medium	0.26
Oranges	1 small	0.24
Parsley	½ cup	5.50
Peas, Green	1 cup	4.00
Potatoes, White	1 medium	0.06
Potatoes, Sweet	1 small	4.00
Rice, Brown	1 cup cooked	2.40
Rye	½ cup	3.00
Soybean Oil	2 tablespoons	46.00
Sunflower Seeds, Raw	½ cup	31.00
Wheatgerm Oil	2 tablespoons	140.00

Plus E's in seeds, raw nuts, spinach, broccoli, avocados, etc. also in cooked beans.

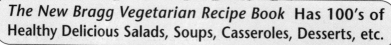

The New Bragg Vegetarian Recipe Book Has 100's of Healthy Delicious Salads, Soups, Casseroles, Desserts, etc.

Latest National Cancer Institute Research and Studies show Vitamin E and improving nutrition reduces cancer risk rates. (www.cancer.gov)

Chapter 16

Doctor Natural Foods

Vitamin E – Nature's Health Miracle

My father and I have found this to be true among the athletes we supervised. For example, Murray Rose, the youngest Olympic triple gold medal winner in history, who eventually won six Olympic medals in distance swimming – took 400 IUs of vitamin E daily and increased it to 1500 IUs during competition. Wheat germ, a prime source of vitamin E, is also an integral part of the training of most top athletes.

Many decades ago when my health pioneer father first introduced the important need for wheat germ and vitamin E supplements to America, he was called a *faddist.* (Paul C. Bragg gave Viobin it's start, today the world's largest wheat germ company.) It's gratifying that today, in these turbulent health care times, his health teachings have finally been substantiated by worldwide scientific research, both laboratory and clinical, in the fields of biochemistry, exercise, nutrition, water and medicine.

Finally people realized that they rob themselves of the *staff of life – vitamin E* when they make bread from refined white flour (*staff of death*). It's tragic that it took over 80 years and caused millions needless premature deaths and overall health deterioration throughout America and worldwide. White flour has been stripped of its precious wheat germ, nature's best source of vitamin E. Everyone who tries to live on the modern civilized diet with refined white flour products devoid of whole grains, suffers from vitamin E deficiency. This has ill effects on people of all ages. Widespread vitamin E deficiency is the prime factor in the disastrous increase in cardiovascular problems, strokes, heart attacks, cancer and illness.

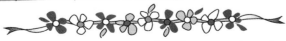

A recent revealing study of 87,000 female nurses whose daily intake of vitamin E was 100 IUs and more showed they had a 40% lower risk of heart attack & stroke than those who did not take vitamin E.

Vitamin E – Your Cardiovascular's Guardian

Pioneer brothers Dr. Evan Shute and Dr. Wilfrid Shute, at their Shute Institute in London, Ontario, Canada, conducted thorough clinical research for over 30 years. They treated over 30,000 cardiovascular patients with high doses of natural source vitamin E with amazing success. Their extensive research on vitamin E has been confirmed, contributed to and furthered by thousands of doctors and biochemists worldwide.

Primary function of vitamin E in the body is to regulate and maintain the health of the entire cardiovascular system. Vitamin E also plays a vital role in the body's defense against air pollution. It also helps to conserve oxygen within the body's cells and blood. The possibility of using vitamin E as an *antidote to smog* has been researched by Dr. Al L. Tappel, Professor of Biochemistry at the University of California, Davis. He believes the natural antioxidation property of vitamin E helps reverse the ageing process. He recommends vitamin E supplements for everyone to help promote a healthier, longer life. *For more suggestions on natural supplements read pages 31, 80, 95, 99, 156.*

This oxygen conserving ability of vitamin E may also be effective in the relief or control of emphysema, the deadly disease of lung deterioration which has increased as our air has become more contaminated. Another healing gift of vitamin E and it's oil or salve is an amazingly effective skin treatment for home application to minor burns, sunburn, skin rashes, scars, and even stretch marks.

Natural vitamin E (*mixed d-alpha tocopherols*) supplements are available at health stores. If just starting on vitamin E, doctors recommend you begin with only 100 IUs daily. Gradually increase to 800 IUs for women and 1200 IUs for men. Raw wheat germ flakes (vacuum packed) and its oil are also good natural sources and available at health stores. Refrigerate both after opening!

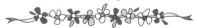

Whole grain products are excellent sources of vit.E, magnesium, selenium and vital elements for maintaining healthy heart and bones. Studies found over 80% of nutrients are lost in refining grains into white flour!

Add Wonder-Working Vitamin E

Raw wheat germ (high in vitamin E) perishes easily. That is why it is refined out of white flour. Apparently commercial millers are more interested in the shelf life of their product, than in the length of your life.

In the Bragg household, we often sprinkle raw wheat germ over our raw vegetable salads, potatoes, vegetables, soups, etc. It has a pleasant, nutty taste. If you like the taste of wheat germ oil (some do, some don't), you will enjoy adding some to your salad dressing. Parents can even add wheat germ oil to the baby's soy, nut or Rice Dream milk. Hollywood actor Clint Eastwood's children thrived on wheat germ oil added to their goat's milk (¼ tsp per cup) after they were weaned at one year.

When you are buying bread, be sure to select only 100% whole grain bread. Better yet, bake your own. We try to bake a delicious variety of breads once a week. Try the healthy, delicious recipes in the Bragg Vegetarian Recipe Book. (See back pages for booklist.)

Another good food source of vitamin E and nutrients is cornmeal mush, made with organic stoneground yellow cornmeal from health stores (not the refined, degerminated variety found in commercial food stores).

Bragg Family's Favorite Cornmeal Recipe

Cup organic cornmeal yellow stoneground
3 to 3½ cups distilled water
3 Tbsps raisins (optional)

Moisten meal with ½ cup cold water. Boil balance of water, then slowly add moistened cornmeal and raisins. Mix well. When evenly thickened, place in top of double boiler (or put pot in pan of water) with low heat so not to burn. Cook 15 minutes. Serve hot. Top with honey, blackstrap molasses, agape nectar or 100% pure maple syrup (our favorite) and sliced fresh fruit (banana, berries, peaches are delicious). Optional topping: Rice Dream & soy non-milks.

Note: If you are serving this to only a few people, there might be some left over. Put it in a flat pan, cool and refrigerate. For breakfast or a main meal, slice and dip in egg (use fertile, free range) batter and roll in wheat germ. Lightly sauté in soy oil. Serve hot. Delicious topped with 100% maple syrup.

Nature's Miracle Phytochemicals Help Prevent Cancer:

Make sure to get your daily dose of these naturally occurring, cancer-fighting biological phytochemicals that are found in fruits, vegetables, grains, legumes, and seeds. They are especially abundant in apples, tomatoes, onions, garlic, beans, legumes, soybeans, cabbage, cauliflower, broccoli, citrus fruits, etc. The champions with the highest count of phytochemicals go to apples and tomatoes.

Class	Food Sources	Action
PHYTOESTROGENS ISOFLAVINS	Soy products, flaxseed, seeds & nuts, yams alfalfa & red clover sprouts, licorice root (not candy)	May block some cancers, & aids in menopausal symptoms and helps improve the memory
PHYTOSTEROLS	Plant oils, corn, flax, pumpkin, sesame, soy, safflower, wheat	Blocks hormonal role in cancers, inhibits uptake of cholesterol from diet
SAPONINS	Yams, beets, beans, cabbage, nuts, soybeans	May prevent cancer cells from multiplying
TERPENES	Carrots, yams, winter squash, sweet potatoes, apples, cantaloupes	Antioxidants – protects DNA from free radical-induced damage
	Tomatoes and tomato-based products	Helps block UVA & UVB & may help protect against cancers, prostate, etc.
	Citrus fruits (flavonoids), apples (quercetin)	Promotes protective enzymes; antiseptic
	Spinach, kale, beet & turnip greens, cabbage	Protects eyes from macular degeneration
	Red chile peppers	Keeps carcinogens from binding to DNA
PHENOLS	Fennel, parsley, carrots, alfalfa, cabbage, apples	Prevents blood clotting & may have anticancer properties
	Citrus fruits, broccoli, cabbage, cucumbers, green peppers, tomatoes	Antioxidants – flavonoids block membrane receptor sites for certain hormones
	Grape seeds, apples	Strong antioxidants; fights germs & bacteria, strengthens immune system, veins & capillaries
	Grapes, especially skins	Antioxidant, antimutagen; promotes detoxification. Acts as carcinogen inhibitors
	Yellow & green squash	Antihepatoxic, antitumor
SULFUR COMPOUNDS	Onions & garlic (fresh is best - we eat both daily. - Patricia Bragg)	Promotes liver enzymes, inhibits cholesterol synthesis, reduces triglycerides, lowers blood pressure, improves immune response, fights infections, germs & parasites

Healthy Eating Gives You More Super Oxygen, Energy and Health

Organic vegetables, fruits and grains are rich in nutrients and vitamin E and contain large amounts of life-giving oxygen. Their juices are very rich in oxygen and distilled water – Mother Nature's purest liquid!

Unsaturated oils – preferably cold or expeller pressed – are exceptionally rich in vitamin E. Combine oil (olive, safflower, soy, flax) with fresh lemon or orange juice or Bragg Organic Raw Apple Cider Vinegar and Bragg Liquid Aminos as a health dressing for salads. (Recipe page 106)

Organic green leafy vegetables also supply organic iron, copper and other important vital minerals that are needed to manufacture hemoglobin in red blood cells. These enable the blood to absorb oxygen from the lungs and transport it to every part of your entire body.

Raw wheat germ, besides supplying the body with vitamin E, is also an important source of organic iron and copper. Other good sources for these minerals are blackberries, blackstrap molasses, dried unsulphured apricots, raw nuts and seeds, dandelion greens, kale, dates, and fertile free-range egg yolks.

Some cooked foods (grains, legumes, vegetables, etc.) enhance a naturally well-balanced diet. Cooking can reduce, in some cases and may even eliminate the vitamin content. Don't overcook! We suggest you lightly steam, bake, broil, stir-fry or wok foods that need cooking.

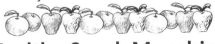

Healthy Snack Munching

Teenagers do a lot of their snacking and eating away from home, buying food from vending machines, fast-food outlets and shopping mall food courts. Armed with the right health info they can easily select and be satisfied with healthy choices; whole fruits, whole grain – honey bakery items rather than high-fat, sugared, white flour snacks that are mostly void of nutrition, plus are harmful to one's health!

The greatest tragedy that comes to man is the emotional depression, the dulling of the intellect and the loss of initiative that comes from nutritive failure. – Dr. James S. McLester, Former President A.M.A.

The Bragg Healthy Lifestyle Promotes Super Health and Super Energy!

When you eat according to The Bragg Healthy Lifestyle, 60% to 70% of your diet will consist of fresh, raw, live foods (organic is best): Raw vegetables, salads, fresh fruits and juices, sprouts, raw seeds & nuts. Enjoy 100% whole grain breads (home-baked is best), whole grain pastas & cereals, organic brown rice, beans & legumes. You can make healthy & delicious combination salads, soups, casseroles, etc., and the nutritious blender drinks that people of all ages will love. These are the healthy, no cholesterol, low-sodium live foods which provide good body fuel for more increased health and vitality. These wholesome foods make joyous, healthy, energized people!

Following The Bragg Healthy Lifestyle, you will become revitalized and reborn into a fresh new life filled with joy, vitality, youthfulness and longevity! There are millions of healthy Bragg followers around the world who have proven to themselves that this Healthy Lifestyle works miracles when followed faithfully.

For more info on the lifestyle that keeps you ageless, read the book *Bragg Healthy Lifestyle – Vital Living to 120!*
(See back pages for Bragg book list information.)

Power Salad for Lunch = Power All Day

Most Americans have schedules which don't permit resting after the midday meal. In Spain, Mexico and many countries worldwide, the main meal is at midday and is followed by a siesta. This short nap is ideal, giving you almost two fresh days in one. Rushed Americans eat their main meal in the evening and then eat a quick, unhealthy meal at noon.

A healthy, large salad of raw fruits or raw garden vegetables (organically grown is best) with raw nuts, sunflower or sesame seeds, soy or feta goats cheese for protein is an ideal delicious luncheon. Try our favorite Bragg Salad and Salad Dressing Recipes on page 106.

The #1 food I recommend is Bragg's organic, raw apple cider vinegar to maintain the body's vital pH acid-alkaline balance. – Gabriel Cousens, M.D.

Vegetarian Protein % Chart

LEGUMES	%
Soybean Sprouts	54
Soybean Curd (tofu)	43
Soy flour	35
Soybeans	35
Broad Beans	32
Lentils	29
Split Peas	28
Kidney Beans	26
Navy Beans	26
Lima Beans	26
Garbanzo Beans	23

VEGETABLES	%
Spirulina (*Plant Algae*)	60
Spinach	49
New Zealand Spinach	47
Watercress	46
Kale	45
Broccoli	45
Brussels Sprouts	44
Turnip Greens	43
Collards	43
Cauliflower	40
Mustard Greens	39
Mushrooms	38
Chinese Cabbage	34
Parsley	34
Lettuce	34
Green Peas	30
Zucchini	28
Green Beans	26
Cucumbers	24
Dandelion Greens	24
Green Pepper	22
Artichokes	22
Cabbage	22
Celery	21
Eggplant	21
Tomatoes	18
Onions	16
Beets	15
Pumpkin	12
Potatoes	11
Yams	8
Sweet Potatoes	6

GRAINS	%
Wheat Germ	31
Rye	20
Wheat, hard red	17
Wild rice	16
Buckwheat	15
Oatmeal	15
Millet	12
Barley	11
Brown Rice	8

FRUITS	%
Lemons	16
Honeydew Melon	10
Cantaloupe	9
Strawberry	8
Orange	8
Blackberry	8
Cherry	8
Apricot	8
Grape	8
Watermelon	8
Tangerine	7
Papaya	6
Peach	6
Pear	5
Banana	5
Grapefruit	5
Pineapple	3
Apple	1

NUTS AND SEEDS	%
Pumpkin Seeds	21
Sunflower Seeds	17
Walnuts, black	13
Sesame Seeds	13
Almonds	12
Cashews	12
Macadamias	9

Data obtained from Nutritive Value of American Foods in Common Units, USDA Agriculture Handbook No. 456. Reprinted with author's permission, from *Diet for a New America* by John Robbins (Walpole, NH: Stillpoint Publishing)

Your Fountain of Youth
Earn Your Bragging Rights with Bragg Healthy Lifestyle

Once you're dedicated to staying healthy and fit, you're living The Bragg Healthy Lifestyle - which can be your Fountain of Youth! By eating and staying healthy, soon you will look forward to your daily exercises as fun and play times - even on the most difficult of days. So plan, plot and follow through with exercising and the Bragg Super Power Breathing Exercises – practice them faithfully throughout the day when time allows.

Put together an exercise routine to do at certain times during the day. You might try a "greet-the-morning" routine upon awakening, then a 10 minute mid-afternoon exercise break for stretching, deep-breathing and stationary jogging. Add longer "shake-off-the-workday" routine that will pep up your circulation and get you ready for an enjoyable evening. Please be faithful – the important thing is to get started – now!!!

Take it from us - once you decide to make exercise a daily habit and get started with it, you won't understand why you ever fought it! After all, who wants to be like the "*do nothing*" man of James Albery's poem? . . .

He slept beneath the moon, basked beneath the sun and
lived a life of going-to-do, and died with nothing done.

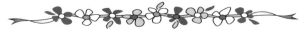

Ponce de Leon

Searched for the "Fountain of Youth."
If he had only known
It's within us . . .
Created by the air we breathe,
the water we drink and food we eat!
Food and drink can make or
Break your health!

Gently forced into action, most lungs will slowly rebuild themselves.
– Basic Physiology

Life is learning which rules to obey, which rules not to obey,
and the wisdom to tell the difference between the two!

104

Chapter 17

Healthy Schedule of 12 Meals Per Week

Eating for Super Health and Longevity

Natural nutrition and correct breathing habits together will lift you to higher levels of vibration for happy, healthful living. To attain and maintain the peak of Super Health, we practice and recommend eating two balanced, healthy meals per day and taking a 24 to 32 hour distilled water fast each week. (Read pages 117, 120).

Upon arising, before our Super Power Breathing exercises, we drink the Bragg Apple Cider Vinegar Drink: 1 to 2 tsps equally of ACV and raw honey (optional) in glass of pure distilled water. Read the Bragg *Apple Cider Vinegar – Miracle Health System* for more info on the miracle uses – page 151.

After our breathing exercises we try to get from one to three hours of outdoor exercise: brisk walking, biking, swimming, hiking, weightlifting, gardening. Then we have some fresh fruit or the Bragg Pep Drink before we get to work; writing, doing radio talk shows by phone, etc.

Our first real meal comes about mid-day. This gives the stomach a thorough rest of 16 to 18 hours, allowing it time to completely empty, recuperate and accumulate an abundant supply of digestive juices after previous evening's meal. <u>Relax and chew each mouthful of food thoroughly</u> *(remember stomachs have no teeth)* <u>so the digestive process will get off to a good start and your food will be assimilated to give you the health and energy you need.</u>

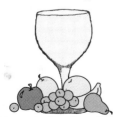

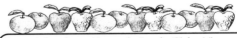

Do as I do – have Bragg's Apple Cider Vinegar drinks daily. 2 tsps Bragg Vinegar & 2 tsps raw honey in 8oz. glass of distilled water. –Julian Witaker, M.D., *www.DrWhitaker.com*

Many studies show that the average overweight American diets three times a year in an effort to lose excess weight, often going on expensive reducing programs, when all they have to do is to follow The Bragg Healthy Lifestyle!

Bragg Lentil & Brown Rice Casserole, Burgers or Soup
Jack LaLanne's Favorite Recipe

14 oz pkg lentils, uncooked	*1½ cups brown organic rice, uncooked*
4 - 6 carrots, chop 1" rounds	*4 garlic cloves, chop, (optional)*
3 celery stalks, chop, (optional)	*1 tsp Bragg Liquid Aminos*
2 onions, chop, (optional)	*¼ tsp Bragg Sprinkle (herbs & spices)*
2-3 quarts, distilled water	*2 tsps Bragg Organic Extra Virgin Olive Oil*

Wash & drain lentils & rice. Place grains in large stainless steel pot. Add water, bring to boil, reduce heat, then add vegetables & seasonings to grains and simmer for 30 minutes. If desired, last 5 minutes add fresh or canned (salt-free) tomatoes before serving. For delicious garnish add spray of Bragg Aminos, minced parsley & nutritional yeast (large) flakes. Mash or blend for burgers. For soup, add more water. Serves 4 to 6.

Bragg Raw Organic Vegetable Health Salad

2 stalks celery, chop	*½ cup alfalfa or sunflower sprouts*
1 bell pepper & seeds, dice	*2 spring onions & green tops, chop*
½ cucumber, slice	*1 raw beet grate*
2 carrots, grate	*1 turnip, grate*
1 cup green cabbage, chop	*1 avocado (ripe)*
½ cup red cabbage, chop	*3 tomatoes, medium size*

For variety add organic raw zucchini, sugar peas, mushrooms, broccoli, cauliflower, (try black olives & pasta). Chop, slice or grate vegetables fine to medium for variety in size. Mix vegetables & serve on bed of lettuce, spinach, watercress or chopped cabbage. Dice avocado & tomato & serve on side as a dressing. Serve choice of fresh squeezed lemon, orange or dressing separately. Chill salad plates before serving. **It's best to always eat salad first before serving hot dishes.** Serves 3 to 5.

Bragg Health Salad Dressing

½ cup Bragg Organic Apple Cider Vinegar   *½ tsp Bragg Liquid Aminos*
1 tsp organic raw honey or agave nectar   *1-2 cloves garlic, mince*
⅓ cup Bragg Organic Olive Oil, or blend with safflower, soy, sesame or flax oil
1 Tbsp fresh herbs, minced or pinch of Bragg Sprinkle (herbs & spices seasoning).

Blend ingredients in blender or jar. Refrigerate in covered jar.

FOR DELICIOUS HERBAL VINEGAR: In quart jar add ⅓ cup tightly packed, crushed fresh sweet basil, tarragon, dill, oregano, or any fresh herbs desired, combined or singly. (If *dried* herbs, use 1-2 tsps. herbs.) Now cover to top with Bragg Vinegar and store two weeks in warm place, and then strain and refrigerate. Also fun to try varieties.

Honey – Celery Seed Vinaigrette

1 tsp Celery Seed	*1 cup Bragg Organic Apple Cider Vinegar*
¼ tsp dry Mustard (optional)	*⅓ cup Bragg Organic Extra Virgin Olive Oil*
½ tsp Bragg Liquid Aminos	*½ tsp peeled fresh Ginger, grate or crush*
⅓ cup raw Honey or to taste	*⅓ tsp Bragg Sprinkle (herbs & spices)*

Blend ingredients in blender or jar. Refrigerate in covered jar.

Enjoy Healthy, Balanced Variety for Dinner

Relax at day's end with some Super Power Breaths. Cleanse the toxins from your lungs so that you will get the full benefit from a well-balanced, nourishing and tasty dinner! Your basic health menu should include:

Salad: A smaller serving this time of fresh raw vegetables and salad greens or try one of these suggestions:

- grated red and green cabbage with diced red and green bell peppers and grated carrots
- grated carrots, sliced raw apples and raisins or try grated carrots, pineapple and raisins
- lettuce, tomato and cucumber salad

See previous page for salad dressing recipes. Sometimes we just squeeze a fresh orange or lemon over our salad and spray Bragg Aminos and Sprinkle over top – it's delicious!

Cooked Vegetables: Include green and yellow veggies; lightly cook, steam, bake, wok or stir-fry. Season with Bragg Aminos for taste delights. We don't add salt!

Protein Dish: Vegetable proteins include all beans, brown rice, lentils, tofu, etc., and all raw, unsalted nuts and seeds (sunflower, pumpkin, sesame, etc.). We strongly recommend a vegetarian diet. If you do eat meat, restrict it to not more than three times a week as a transition on the way to your vegetarian diet. N*ever add table salt!* Prepare your foods with healthy, nutritious flavors from fresh garlic, onions, lemon juice, herbs and delicious Bragg Liquid Aminos which is made from only, pure certified non GMO healthy soy beans.

Dessert: If eaten, it should be fresh fruit when available, or unsweetened, honey-stewed or dried fruit. For special desserts make one of the healthy pies, cakes, cookies, etc., in the *Bragg Vegetarian Health Recipe Book*.

Beverages: For health, it's best not to drink beverages with meals, not even water! Your digestive juices do their best work undiluted. Have ample fluids hour before and hour after meals and during daytime. At least an hour after dinner, you may have the delicious Bragg Apple Cider Drink (hot or cold), herbal tea or a glass of fresh fruit or vegetable juice, if you wish. Drink all the distilled water you want between meals–ideal is 8 glasses daily!

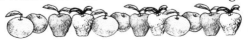

*Enjoy healthy, organic foods for their
wonderful abundance of life energy.*

Eliminating Meat is Safer and Healthier

Play it safe, become a healthy vegetarian. They feed cattle antibiotics, growth hormones and the dead, ground up carcasses of other feed lot animals who didn't make it to the slaughterhouse. See web: earthsave.org.

What kind of chemical reaction would occur in your body if somebody put a choke chain around your neck to keep you in line, shoved you onto a conveyor belt, and made you watch in horror as all of those in line in front of you were beheaded one by one? Your body would be pumped full of <u>adrenaline from all that fear</u>! <u>Unused adrenaline is extremely toxic</u>. If you think for a minute that most of the meat that you consume is not packed with this toxic substance, you're sadly mistaken!

Also, consider the fact that cattle, sheep, chickens, etc., are all vegetarians by nature. When you eat them, you are just eating polluted vegetables. Why not skip all the waste and toxins and just eat healthy, organic vegetables?

Meat is also a major source of cholesterol and uric acid, both harmful to your health. If you are going to include <u>meat in your diet, it should not be eaten more than three times a week</u>. In our opinion, fresh fish can be the least toxic of the flesh proteins. Beware of fish from polluted waters, they can be contaminated with mercury, lead, cadmium, dangerous pesticides and many other toxic substances. If you are unable to test the waters from where your fish come, don't risk eating them. <u>And avoid shellfish – shrimp, lobster and crayfish. They are garbage-eating bottom-feeders – the rats and flies of the water kingdom</u>. They eat the rotting, decaying scum and refuse off the bottoms of the oceans, lakes and rivers. Next comes chicken and turkey. Don't eat the skin, it's heavy in cholesterol. Third place goes to lamb and beef. More shocking facts follow.

<u>People should not eat pork or pork products of any kind. The pig is the only animal besides man that develops arteriosclerosis or hardening of the arteries. In fact, this animal is so loaded with cholesterol that in cold weather, unprotected pigs and hogs will become</u>

solid and stiff, as though frozen solid and some die. This animal is also often infected with a dangerous parasite which causes the disease called trichinosis.

And what about that myth that you have to eat meat to get your protein? If that were true, where do you suppose farm animals, especially work horses and fast race horses get their protein? They are vegetarians! They get their protein from the grains and grasses that they eat. You are no different. You can get the proteins you need from the large variety of whole grains, beans, raw nuts, seeds, beans, fruits and vegetables that God put on this planet for your health and enjoyment.

We enjoy being vegetarians and not polluting our bodies with unhealthy meat, fowl and fish proteins. We feel it's safer and healthier getting our proteins from organic vegetables, sprouts, beans, brown rice, legumes, nuts, seeds, etc. See Vegetable Protein % Chart, page 103.

Do Not Poison Your Body with Toxic, Foodless Foods and Harmful Drinks!

In our industrialized, urbanized civilization, we pay a heavy price for the convenience of mass distribution of foodstuffs. Not only has our flour been bleached and robbed of its vital wheat germ, but the majority of commercial foods have been devitalized, demineralized – rendered *foodless* – in order to give them a longer *shelf life.* You are risking your own life when you eat these *foodless foods* that cannot nourish your body properly. Many contain preservatives and additives (such as nitrates and nitrites) whose cumulative effect has proven to be extremely harmful to the human body.

Even though the Federal Food & Drug Administration (FDA) requires the listing of most ingredients on processed, packaged and canned foods, few people bother to read the fine print. If they do, they rarely understand it or take the trouble to find out what the various additives are and what effect they have on the human body. You don't have to be a chemist to find the answers; just look in a modern dictionary.

Avoid All Dangerous Embalmers – Preservatives

For example, *Webster's Dictionary* defines *nitrate* as a *"salt or ester of nitric acid"* and defines *nitric acid* as a *"corrosive liquid inorganic acid HNO₃"*. Ordinary common sense can figure out what a steady diet of toxic foods containing a concentrated form of a corrosive liquid inorganic acid will do to your body! Nitrates and nitrites are deadly preservatives. Avoid them like the plague!

Sulphur dioxide is another commercial preservative commonly used on dried fruits. It is defined by Webster as a *"heavy pungent gas, easily condensed to a colorless liquid and used especially in making sulfuric acid."* Do we have to remind you that <u>sulfuric acid eats away flesh</u>?

Many natural fats and oils are ruined by *hydrogenation.* This hardening process keeps them from becoming rancid, but renders them absolutely indigestible and causes terrible clogging of the cardiovascular system. Read all labels and understand them! Stop eating all commercially refined and processed foods made with refined white flour, refined white sugar, processed *lunch meats* and cheeses and foods with hydrogenated fats, harmful additives and preservatives such as sodium nitrate, MSG (monosodium glutamate), sulfur dioxide, etc.

Although they are not labeled *poison,* coffee, tea and alcohol should be banished from your diet! Why? Because their harmful ingredients accumulate poisons in your body. Also avoid soft drinks and cola drinks. They contain toxic fluoridated water, artificial flavors, colors, preservatives and sweeteners. They will poison your bloodstream and body. The huge quantities of phosphorus in soda depletes calcium and magnesium from the body. Result: millions suffer with osteoporosis.

Salt was the first food preservative discovered by man. It has been used for thousands of years by humans who erroneously believed salt a necessity of life. Cultures unexposed to the western culture often don't use added salt in their native diets. <u>They stay remarkably healthy until introduced to the western diet poisons</u>. Then their deterioration is rapid and tragic. My father and I have seen this happen from Africa to the Arctic; especially the South Sea islands, Hawaii, Samoa and Tahiti.

Caution Using Salt – It's a Slow Killer!
We can't stress it enough: Avoid using salt!

The *salt of the earth* (inorganic sodium chloride) is poisonous to humans, plants and animals. What about *salt licks?* Don't even wild animals crave salt? My father investigated this thoroughly – and found that salt licks never contain sodium chloride. They are decomposed plant life made into organic minerals. The commercial salt licks used by cattle ranchers are to make the cattle thirsty so that they will drink volumes of water and therefore weigh more when they are ready to be sold. This is why meat *shrinks* excessively when cooked.

All animals, including man, need organic minerals. Only plants can digest inorganic minerals, which they take from the earth and convert through photosynthesis into organic minerals to feed the animal kingdom. This is Mother Nature's and God's marvelous balance.

Our ancestors discovered that salt (inorganic sodium chloride) would preserve meat from decay. Remember, they had no refrigeration or means of storing food for long periods. Because their lifestyles were extremely active, their bodies could eliminate this indigestible salt, an inorganic mineral that plays havoc in the body.

Most civilized people over 40, today are basically sedentary creatures. Most cannot eliminate or assimilate the excessive amount of salt they consume. Their bodies stash it away in crystals that harden in the lining of their arteries and other blood vessels and in their joints, feet and hands, etc. causing arthritis and pain. Some of the salt is stored in a water solution that bloats the tissues. This can cause congestive heart failure and even death. Eliminate salt from your diet! If you think your food tastes *flat* without it, add Bragg Liquid Aminos, Bragg Sea Kelp, or our delicious organic herb – spice seasoning Bragg Sprinkle, a 50 year favorite that is now available again. Take a lesson from famous French chefs, who use very little or no salt! They achieve marvelous flavors by skillful use of herbs, garlic, onions and mushrooms. Also vinegar and lemon juice are good seasoners for salads, veggies, beans, rice, legumes and other foods.

Salt actually deadens your taste buds. Stay away from salt. Your taste buds will awaken and you will soon start to enjoy the natural flavors of the foods you eat. Even more importantly, you will become healthier and live longer when you give up salt and live a healthy life!

8 Glasses Pure Water – Essential for Health!

Distilled water is the world's purest and best water! It's excellent for detoxification and fasting programs because it helps cleanse and flush toxins and harmful substances out of the cells, organs and fluids of the body!

Most water from chemically-treated (toxic fluorides, chlorides, etc.) public water systems, and even some wells and springs, most likely contain harmful chemicals and toxic elements. Too often the water in our homes, offices, schools, hospitals, etc., are loaded with toxins; zinc, copper, cadmium or even lead from old soldered pipes.

The pure water from the fresh juices of vegetables, fruits and other foods, or the clean rain (distilled) water or steam (bottled) distilled water is essential for super health. Your body is constantly working for you. It's 70% water and the liquids you put in it will either nourish you or harm you and may even eventually kill you!

Your body breaks down old bone and tissue cells and replaces them with new ones. As your body casts off old minerals and the broken-down cells, it must obtain new supplies of the essential elements in order to make healthy, new cells. (Important reason to eat healthy foods.)

Scientists discovered that many disorders, including dental problems, different types of arthritis, osteoporosis and some forms of hardening of the arteries are in part due to imbalances in the levels and ratios of minerals in the body. Every body requires a proper balance of all the nutritive elements in order to remain healthy. It's as bad for a person to have too much of one item as it is to have too little of another. In order for calcium to be able to create new cells of bone and teeth, you must have adequate levels of phosphorus and magnesium. Yet, if there is too much of these minerals or too little calcium, etc. in the diet, old bone will be taken away, but new bone will not be formed. Read more info page 156.

High Protein Diet Depletes Minerals

Unbalanced and unhealthy diets can deplete the body of calcium, magnesium, potassium and other major elements. (See page 156.) Diets high in proteins, meats, fish, eggs and grains may provide excesses of phosphorus which deplete calcium and magnesium from the bones and tissues. This causes these minerals to be lost in the urine. High fat diets tend to increase the uptake of phosphorus from the intestines relative to calcium and other basic minerals. This can produce losses of calcium, magnesium, etc. like the high phosphorus diet, sodas, etc.

Deficiencies of calcium and magnesium can produce many different health problems, from osteoporosis to muscular cramping, hyperactivity, muscular twitching, (crazy leg syndrome), sleep disorders and frequency of urination. Deficiencies or imbalances of other minerals can produce many other health problems.

It is very important to clean and detoxify the body through fasting and by drinking 8 glasses pure distilled water and organically grown vegetable and fruit juices. In order to continually provide the body with new supplies of minerals, adults need a diet containing a variety of organic vegetables, also mineral rich kelp and other sea vegetables. Also infants need healthy mother's milk preferably to one year of age for solid foundation!

Many adults and children in western civilizations are malnourished and have low levels of essential minerals in their bodies due to losses caused by coffee, tea, cola and carbonated beverages and processed foods and modern diets containing refined sugar, flours and salt.

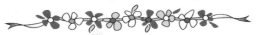

A wise man should consider that health is the greatest of human blessings and learn how, by his own thought, to derive benefit from his illnesses. Change any unhealthy living habits to 100% healthy habits and start now!

Remember your body needs lots of water, if bowels & kidneys are to function normally. If you use laxatives or diuretics, water and herbals are gentler. Gradually increase your water intake to 8 glasses of distilled water to fight dehydration.

Nature never deceives us; it's always we who deceive ourselves.– Rousseau

Open your mind, for the doors of wisdom are never shut. – Ben Franklin

The body's organ systems can become unbalanced by chronic stress; by toxins in our air, water and soil; by disease-produced injuries; in babies, by the prenatal nutritional deficiencies in the mother's diet; and their unhealthy lifestyle habits. Thus, people in our fast-food society need to take a natural multi-vitamin and mineral food supplement to ensure they get their vital nutrients. We suggest everyone take them for extra protection.

Fast One Day Each Week for Inner Cleansing

Oxygen, as we have stressed, is the greatest cleanser and purifier of the body. Give it a chance to do a thorough house cleansing: help your body rid itself of accumulated toxic poisons by going on a 24 to 36 hour fast every week. Monday is our favorite fast day.

During this fast, drink 8-10 glasses of distilled water daily. Three flavor with fresh lemon juice or 1-2 tsps Bragg Organic Raw Apple Cider Vinegar with (optional) 1-2 tsps honey, agave nectar or maple syrup to taste (diabetics use Stevia). Some add pinch of cayenne. No food, juices or supplements are necessary. Some start with juice fasts pages 117-118. If you want a warm drink, have herbal tea or delicious hot Bragg Liquid Aminos Broth (1tsp in cup hot water) or Bragg Vinegar Drink (see recipes page 116).

When freed from the daily chore of digesting and assimilating food, your body will use its oxygen-sparked energy to do a more thorough internal cleansing. After your first fast you will feel a renewed vitality. Make this a weekly habit and, as time goes on, you will feel even more invigorated and rejuvenated. *Life is precious - Patricia Bragg*

Monday is our regular weekly fast day. After our evening meal on Sunday, we take nothing but 8 to 10 glasses of distilled water until Tuesday morning. We have been doing this fast in the Bragg family for the last 90 years and are all living healthy, long lives. We also try to fast for the first three days of each month.

Several times each year we take a longer fast of 7 to 10 days. Our favorite fast is distilled water for a week. It works wonders in keeping us fit and trim. If you would like to know more about the methods and benefits of fasting, consult our Bragg book, *The Miracle of Fasting.* Read page 120. (This book has changed the lives of millions worldwide. It's been #1 in Russia and Ukraine for over 18 years.)

Distilled Water is the #1 Health Drink

Not merely on fast days, but every day of your life, let the water you drink be pure distilled water. You'll be *drinking oxygen* with this pure H_2O! As well as fresh fruit and vegetable juices – which are naturally distilled – this is the only *safe* water to drink on our polluted planet.

Even rain water – which is naturally distilled water when it leaves the clouds – is contaminated if it passes through a heavily polluted atmosphere. (We love the smell of rain-washed air.) Mineral water and ground water (from springs, wells, streams, etc.) contain inorganic minerals which cannot be assimilated by the body and which can collect in the body and produce harmful deposits in the blood vessels, joints, kidneys and gallbladder. Water from reservoirs chemically treated to kill germs contains inorganic minerals and harsh chemicals (toxic chlorine, etc.) that are very harmful to the body! Don't drink water treated by water softeners! It contains suspended inorganic minerals that produce more *suds* ideal for washing clothes and dishes; but this chemically softened water is harmful to your body.

Use distilled water for drinking and cooking to ensure a longer life and health for you and your family! You will find the complete, documented report on the health hazards of chemicalized, fluoride, waters and reasons for drinking only pure distilled water in our book, *Water – The Shocking Truth!* (See booklist back pages of this book).

Keep Fluoride Out of Your Water!

Most of the water that Americans drink has fluoride in it, including tap, bottled and canned drinks! Now, the ADA (American Dental Association) is insisting that the FDA mandates the addition of fluoride to all bottled waters! Defend your right to drink pure, non-fluoridated tap and bottled waters! Challenge and stop local and state water fluoridation policies! Call, write, fax or e-mail your state officials, Congressional representatives, and the President!

CHECK FOLLOWING WEBSITES FOR FLUORIDE UPDATES:

- www.fluoridation.com • www.keepersofthewell.org
- www.fluoridealert.org • www.riv.net/–fluoride
- www.fluoride-journal.com • www.bragg.com
- www.bruha.com/fluoride
- www.gjne.com/cfsdwh
- www.nofluoride.com
- www.zerowasteamerica.org/fluoride.htm

fluoride is deadly

HEALTHY BEVERAGES
Fresh Juices, Herb Teas & Pep Drinks

These freshly squeezed organic vegetable and fruit juices are important to The Bragg Healthy Lifestyle. It's not wise to drink beverages with your main meals, as it dilutes the digestive juices. But it's great during the day to have a glass of freshly squeezed orange, grapefruit, vegetable juice, Bragg Vinegar ACV Drink, herb tea or try hot cup Bragg Liquid Aminos Broth (½ to 1 tsp Bragg Liquid Aminos in cup of hot distilled water) – these are all ideal pick-me-up beverages.

Bragg Apple Cider Vinegar Cocktail – Mix 1-2 tsps equally of Bragg Organic ACV and (optional) raw honey, blackstrap molasses, agave nectar or pure maple syrup in 8 oz. distilled or purified water. Take glass upon arising, hour before lunch and dinner (*if diabetic, to sweeten use 2-4 stevia drops*).

Delicious Hot or Cold Cider Drink – Add 2 to 3 cinnamon sticks and 4 cloves to water and boil. Steep 20 minutes or more. Before serving add Bragg Vinegar and raw honey to taste. (*Re-use cinnamon sticks & cloves*)

Bragg Favorite Juice Cocktail – This drink consists of all raw vegetables (please remember organic is best) which we prepare in our vegetable juicer: carrots, celery, beets, cabbage, tomatoes, watercress and parsley, etc. The great purifier garlic, we enjoy but it's optional.

Bragg Favorite Health Smoothie "Pep" Drink – After morning stretch and exercises we often enjoy this drink instead of fruit. It's delicious and powerfully nutritious as a meal anytime: lunch, dinner or take in thermos to work, school, sports, gym, hiking, and to park or freeze for popsicles.

Bragg Health Smoothie "Pep" Drink

Prepare following in blender, add frozen juice cube if desired colder; Choice of: freshly squeezed orange or grapefruit juice; carrot and greens juice; unsweetened pineapple juice; or 1½ - 2 cups purified or distilled water with:

2 tsps spirulina or green powder, barley, etc.	*1 to 2 bananas, ripe*
½ tsp raw wheat germ (optional)	*1 tsp soy protein powder*
½ Tbsp flax oil (or grind Tbsp of flax seeds)	*1 tsp sunflower or chia seeds*
½ tsp lecithin granules	*1 tsp raw honey (optional)*
1 tsp rice or oat bran	*1 tsp vit C or emer'gen-C powder*
½ tsp psyllium husk powder (optional)	*½ tsp nutritional yeast flakes*
2 dates or prunes, pitted (optional)	*⅓ cup soy yogurt or soft tofu*

Optional: 8 apricots (sundried, unsulphured) soak in jar overnight in purified water or unsweetened pineapple juice. We soak enough for several days, keep refrigerated – also delicious topped with soy yogurt . Add seasonal organic fresh fruit: peaches, strawberries, berries, apricots, etc. instead of banana. In winter, add apples, kiwi, oranges, tangelos, persimmons or pears, and if fresh is unavailable, try sugar-free, frozen organic fruits. Servings 1 to 2.

Patricia's Delicious Health Popcorn

Use freshly popped organic popcorn (use air popper). Try Bragg Organic Olive Oil, Flax Oil or melted salt-free butter over popcorn. Add several sprays Bragg Aminos and Bragg Apple Cider Vinegar. . . Yes – it's delicious! Now sprinkle with nutritional yeast (large) flakes. For variety try pinch of Italian or French herbs, Bragg Kelp, Bragg Sprinkle (herb/spices), mustard powder or fresh crushed garlic to oil mixture. It's delicious – serve instead of breads!

Juice Fasting – Introductory Road to Water Fasting

Fasting has been rediscovered through juice fasting as a simply delicious and easy means of cleansing and purifying and rebuilding health and vitality.

To fast (*abstain from food*) is from the Old English word *fasten or to hold firm*. It's a means to commit oneself to the task of finding inner strength through cleansing of the body, mind and soul. Throughout history the world's greatest church leaders, philosophers and sages including Socrates, Plato, Buddha and Gandhi have enjoyed fasting and preached its many miracle benefits.

Juice bars are springing up everywhere and juice fasting has become "in" with the Stars of Hollywood and Broadway. The number of Stars who believe in the miracle power and effectiveness of juice and water fasting is growing. Some are: Steven Spielberg, Barbra Streisand, Kim Basinger, Alec Baldwin, Christie Brinkley, Dolly Parton, Donna Karan, etc., and author Danielle Steel. They say fasting helps balance their lives physically, mentally, spiritually and emotionally.

Although a distilled water fast is best, an introductory liquid juice fast can offer people an opportunity to give their intestinal systems restful, cleansing relief from the commercial, high-fat, sugar, salt, protein and "fast foods" diets. Too many Americans exist daily on diets that cause obesity and illness.

Organic raw live fruit and vegetable juices now are available fresh from health stores and juice bars. You can also prepare these healthy juices yourself using a good home juicer. When juice fasting, it's best to dilute the juice with ⅓ distilled or purified water. This list (page 118) gives you delicious varieties. With vegetable and tomato combinations try adding dash of Bragg Liquid Aminos or Bragg Sprinkle (herbs/spices). Non-fast days, try some of the nutritious green powders (barley, chlorella, spirulina, etc.) to create a powerful health drink. When using herbs in these drinks, use 1 to 2 fresh leaves, mince or a pinch of Bragg Sprinkle or Bragg Kelp Seasoning (seaweed), rich in protein, iodine and iron – is delicious with vegetable juices. *These are also delicious sprinkled on salads, veggies, soups, potatoes, etc.*

Dine with little, sup with less; do better still, sleep supperless. – Ben Franklin

117

Here are Some Powerful Juice Combinations:

1. Beet, celery, alfalfa sprouts
2. Cabbage, celery and apple
3. Cabbage, cucumber, celery, tomato, spinach and basil
4. Tomato, carrot and mint
5. Carrot, celery, watercress, garlic and wheatgrass
6. Grapefruit, orange and lemon
7. Beet, parsley, celery, carrot, kale, mustard greens, garlic
8. Beet, celery, carrot and kelp
9. Cucumber, carrot and parsley
10. Watercress, cucumber, garlic
11. Asparagus, carrot, and mint
12. Carrot, celery, parsley, onion, cabbage and kelp
13. Carrot and coconut milk
14. Carrot, broccoli, lemon, cayenne
15. Carrot, cabbage, rosemary
16. Apple, carrot, radish, ginger
17. Apple, pineapple and mint
18. Apple, papaya and grapes
19. Papaya, cranberries and apple
20. Leafy greens, broccoli, apple
21. Grape, kiwi and apple
22. Watermelon (seeds optional)

Paul C. Bragg Introduced Juicing to America

Juicing has come a long way since my father imported the first hand operated vegetable-fruit juicer from Germany. Before, this juice was pressed by hand using cheesecloth. He introduced his new juice therapy idea, then pineapple juice, then later tomato juice, to the American public. These two juices were erroneously thought to be too acid. Now, these health beverages have become the favorites of millions. TV's famous *Juicemen* Jack LaLanne and Jay Kordich say Bragg was their early inspiration and mentor! They both are ageless and are still going strong, inspiring millions to health.

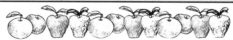

Through our actions and deeds, rather than promises,
let us display the essence of love – perfect harmony in motion!
– Philip Glyn, Welsh Poet

Kindness should be a frame of mind in which we are alert
to every chance to do, to give, to share and to cheer.

Little deeds of kindness, little words of love,
Help to make earth happy, like the Heaven above.
– Julia A. F. Carney

Kindness comes in all sizes.
Sometimes it is only
A little thing we give –
A trifle, a smile, a piece of fruit,
A hug, and a kind word.
If it is given willingly,
The kindness is doubled. – Syrus

Food and Product Summary

Today, many of our foods are highly processed or refined, robbing them of essential nutrients, vitamins, minerals and enzymes. Many also contain harmful, toxic and dangerous chemicals. The research findings and experience of top nutritionists, physicians and dentists have led to the discovery that devitalized foods are a major cause of poor health, illness, cancer and premature death. The enormous increase in the last 80 years of degenerative diseases such as heart disease, arthritis and dental decay substantiate this belief. Scientific research has shown that most of these afflictions can be prevented and that others, once established, can be arrested or even reversed through wise nutritional methods.

Enjoy Super Health with Natural Foods

1. **RAW FOODS:** Fresh fruits and raw vegetables organically grown are always best. Enjoy nutritious variety garden salads with raw vegetables, sprouts, raw nuts and seeds.

2. **VEGETABLES and PROTEINS:**
   a. Legumes, lentils, brown rice, tofu, soy & all beans.
   b. Nuts and seeds, raw and unsalted.
   c. We prefer healthier vegetarian proteins. If you must have animal protein, then be sure it's hormone–free, and organically fed and no more than 1 or 2 times a week.
   d. Dairy products – Organic fed, fertile, range-free eggs, unprocessed hard cheese and feta goat's cheese. We choose not to use dairy products. Try the healthier non-dairy soy, rice, nut, and almond milks and soy cheeses, delicious yogurt and soy and rice ice cream.

3. **FRUITS and VEGETABLES:** Organically grown is always best – grown without the use of poisonous sprays and toxic chemical fertilizers whenever possible; urge your market to stock organic produce! Steam, bake, sauté or wok vegetables as short a time as possible to retain the best nutritional content and flavor. Also enjoy fresh juices.

4. **100% WHOLE GRAIN CEREALS, BREADS and FLOURS:** They contain important B-complex vitamins, vitamin E, minerals, fiber and the important unsaturated fatty acids.

5. **COLD or EXPELLER-PRESSED VEGETABLE OILS:** Bragg organic extra virgin olive oil (is best), soy, sunflower, flax, mac and sesame oils are excellent sources of healthy, essential, unsaturated fatty acids. We use oils sparingly.

USA leads the world in heart disease, strokes, cancer and diabetes! Why? It's our fast junk foods, high sugars, fats, milk and processed foods diet.

119

BENEFITS FROM THE JOYS OF FASTING

Fasting renews your faith in yourself, your strength and Gods strength.
Fasting is easier than any diet. • Fasting is the quickest way to lose weight.
Fasting is adaptable to a busy life. • Fasting gives the body a physiological rest.
Fasting is used successfully in the treatment of many physical illnesses.
Fasting can yield weight losses of up to 10 pounds or more in the first week.
Fasting lowers & normalizes cholesterol, homocysteine & blood pressure levels.
Fasting improves dietary habits. • Fasting increases pleasure eating healthy foods.
Fasting is a calming experience, often relieving tension and insomnia.
Fasting frequently induces feelings of euphoria, a natural high.
Fasting is a miracle rejuvenator, slowing the ageing process.
Fasting is a natural stimulant to rejuvenate the growth hormone levels.
Fasting is an energizer, not a debilitator. • Fasting aids the elimination process.
Fasting often results in a more vigorous marital relationship.
Fasting can eliminate smoking, drug and drinking addictions.
Fasting is a regulator, educating the body to consume food only as needed.
Fasting saves time spent marketing, preparing and eating.
Fasting rids the body of toxins, giving it an internal shower & cleansing.
Fasting does not deprive the body of essential nutrients.
Fasting can be used to uncover the sources of food allergies.
Fasting is used effectively in schizophrenia treatment & other mental illnesses.
Fasting under proper supervision can be tolerated easily up to four weeks.
Fasting does not accumulate appetite; hunger pangs disappear in 1-2 days.
Fasting is routine for the animal kingdom.
Fasting has been a common practice since the beginning of man's existence.
Fasting is a rite in all religions; the Bible alone has 74 references to it.
Fasting under proper conditions is absolutely safe. • Fasting is a blessing.
Fasting is not starving, it's nature's cure that God has given us. – Patricia Bragg
– Allan Cott, M.D., *Fasting As A Way Of Life*

Spiritual Bible Reasons Why We Should Fast

Acts 13:2-3	Deut. 11:7-14,21	Luke 4:2-5,14	Matthew 9: 9-15
Acts 14:23-25	Ezra 8:23	Luke 9:1-6,11	Matthew 17:18-21
3 John 2	Gen. 6:3	Mark 2:16-20	Neh. 1:4
1 Cor. 10:31	Gal. 5:16-26	Matthew 4:1-4	Neh. 9:1, 20-21
1 Cor. 13:4-7	Isaiah 58:6,8	Matthew 6:16-18	Psalms 35:13
Deut. 8:3-8	Joel 2:12	Matthew 7:7-8	Psalms 119:18

Dear Health Friend,

This gentle reminder explains the great benefits from *The Miracle of Fasting* that you will enjoy when starting on your weekly 24 hour Bragg Fasting Program for Super Health! It's a precious time of body-mind-soul cleansing and renewal.

On fast days I drink 8 to 10 glasses of distilled (our favorite) or purified water, (I add 1-2 tsps Bragg Organic Vinegar to 3 of them). If just starting, you may also try herbal teas or diluted fresh juices with ⅓ distilled water. Every day, even some fast days, add 1 Tbsp of psyllium husk powder to liquids once daily. It's an extra cleanser and helps normalize weight, cholesterol and blood pressure and helps promote healthy elimination. Fasting is the oldest, most effective healing method known to man. Fasting offers great, miraculous blessings from Mother Nature and our Creator. It begins the self-cleansing of the inner-body workings so we can promote our own self-healing.

My father and I wrote the book *The Miracle of Fasting* to share with you the health miracles it can perform in your life. It's all so worthwhile to do and it's an important part of The Bragg Healthy Lifestyle.

With Love, *Patricia*

Paul Bragg's work on fasting and water is one of the great contributions to The Healing Wisdom and The Natural Health Movement in the world today.
– Gabriel Cousens, M.D., Author of Conscious Eating & Spiritual Nutrition

Avoid These Processed, Refined, Harmful Foods

Once you realize the harm caused to your body by unhealthy, refined, chemicalized, deficient foods, you'll want to eliminate these "killer" foods. Also avoid microwaved foods! Follow The Bragg Healthy Lifestyle to provide the basic, healthy nourishment to maintain your health.

- Refined sugar, artificial sweeteners (toxic aspartame, splenda) or their products: jams, jellies, preserves, marmalades, yogurts, ice cream, sherbets, Jello, cake, candy, cookies, all chewing gum, colas & diet drinks, pies, pastries, and all sugared fruit juices & fruits canned in sugar syrup. **(Health Stores have healthy delicious replacements, Stevia, Agave Nectar, etc, so seek and buy the best.)**

- White flour products such as white bread, wheat-white bread, enriched flours, rye bread that has white flour in it, dumplings, biscuits, buns, gravy, pasta, pancakes, waffles, soda crackers, pizza, ravioli, pies, pastries, cakes, cookies, prepared and commercial puddings and ready-mix bakery products. Most made with dangerous (oxy-cholesterol) powdered milk and powdered eggs. **(Health Stores have huge variety of 100% whole grain organic products, delicious breads, crackers, pastas, desserts, etc.)**

- Salted foods, such as corn chips, potato chips, pretzels, crackers and nuts.

- Refined white rices and pearled barley. • Fast fried foods. • Indian ghee.

- Refined, sugared (*also aspartame, splenda*), dry processed cereals – cornflakes, etc.

- Foods that contain olestra, palm and coconut oils. These additives are not fit for human consumption and should be totally avoided.

- Peanuts and peanut butter that contain hydrogenated, hardened oils and any peanut mold and all molds that can cause allergies.

- Margarine – combines heart-deadly trans-fatty acids and saturated fats.

- Saturated fats and hydrogenated oils – enemies that clog the arteries.

- Coffee, decaffeinated coffee, caffeinated tea and all alcoholic beverages. Also all caffeinated and sugared water-juices, all cola and soft drinks.

- Fresh pork and products. • Fried, fatty meats. • Irradiated and GMO foods.

- Smoked meats, such as ham, bacon, sausage and smoked fish.

- Luncheon meats, hot dogs, salami, bologna, corned beef, pastrami and packaged meats containing dangerous sodium nitrate or nitrite.

- Dried fruits containing sulphur dioxide – a toxic preservative.

- Don't eat chickens or turkeys that have been injected with hormones or fed with commercial poultry feed containing any drugs or toxins.

- Canned soups - read labels for sugar, salt, starch, flour and preservatives.

- Foods containing benzoate of soda, salt, sugar, and any additives, drugs, preservatives; irradiated and genetically engineered foods.

- Day-old cooked vegetables, potatoes and pre-mixed, wilted lifeless salads.

- All commercial vinegars: pasteurized, filtered, distilled, white, malt and synthetic vinegars are dead vinegars! *(We use only our Bragg Organic Raw, Unfiltered Apple Cider Vinegar with the "Mother Enzyme" as used in olden times.)*

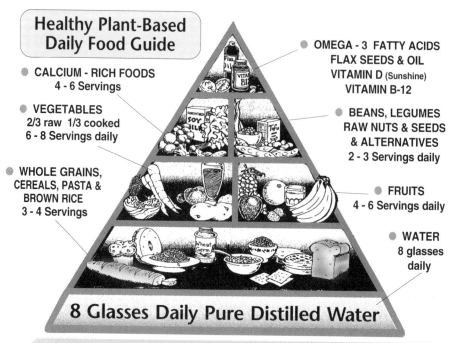

Healthy Plant-Based Daily Food Guide

- **CALCIUM - RICH FOODS**
  4 - 6 Servings

- **VEGETABLES**
  2/3 raw 1/3 cooked
  6 - 8 Servings daily

- **WHOLE GRAINS,
  CEREALS, PASTA &
  BROWN RICE**
  3 - 4 Servings

- **OMEGA - 3 FATTY ACIDS
  FLAX SEEDS & OIL
  VITAMIN D** (Sunshine)
  VITAMIN B-12

- **BEANS, LEGUMES
  RAW NUTS & SEEDS
  & ALTERNATIVES**
  2 - 3 Servings daily

- **FRUITS**
  4 - 6 Servings daily

- **WATER**
  8 glasses
  daily

8 Glasses Daily Pure Distilled Water

Deadly Smog's CA. Cost over $521 M Annually

Los Angeles – California could prevent 3.3 million school absences and 4,000 asthma-related hospital admissions each year by adopting stricter air quality standards currently under consideration by the state Air Resources Board, according to an analysis by an environmental advocacy group.

High ozone levels currently cost $521 million a year in hospital admissions, emergency room visits and missed school days, according to estimates released recently by the Environmental Working Group, which analyzed three years of California's air quality data. The pollution disproportionately affects children and asthma patients, the report said.

The analysis comes one week before the Air Resources Board meets to consider adding a new regulation to limit ozone levels in California's 34 air quality districts. State standards are already tougher than federal ones and the new proposal would tighten those regulations even more, said Gennet Paauwe, a spokesman for the California State Board.

The study estimated that school absences statewide related to smog induced illnesses that cost local school districts $82 million a year in lost state funding because the state ties its funding to attendance numbers. The cost to those children's parents annually tripled that amount, the group estimated. The results are no surprise to many school administrators and teachers. "You ought to see all the inhalers we have here," said Fred Medina, principal at North Elementary School in Tracy, a San Joaquin Valley community. "Our secretaries have to be the nurse and secretary in this office." Mr. Medina said he limits the activities allowed in physical education classes on bad-air days (See pages 92-94).

You are what you breathe, eat, drink, think, say and do! – Patricia Bragg, N.D., Ph.D.

Chapter 18

Powerful Benefits of Bragg Super Power Breathing

A Strong Mind in A Strong Healthy Body

Greek civilization, which produced some of the greatest minds the world has known, lived by the motto: *A strong mind in a strong body.* The Ancient Greeks were noted for their amazing powers of endurance, robust health and youthful longevity. All of these were the results of their systems of natural eating, deep breathing and strenuous exercise, which produced physiques that have served as the models of classical art ever since.

The classic Greeks followed four main health principles:

1. Full deep super power breathing.
2. Eating two meals of natural healthy foods per day.
3. Exercise regime for complete body development.
4. They honored supreme health, body, mind and soul.

We can do the same and achieve the same results they did. We can become more vital and totally fit – enjoying every minute of being alive. The time to start is NOW – whatever your calendar years. Whether you are a teenager or a great-grandparent or somewhere in between, it is never too early or too late to start on the Supreme Road to Super Health!

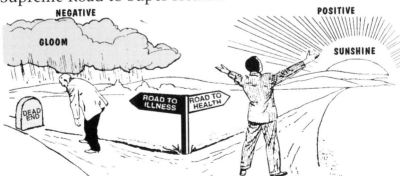

The choice of which road to take is up to the individual. He alone can decide whether he wants to reach a dead end or live a healthy lifestyle for a long, healthy, happy, active life.
– Paul C. Bragg, N.D., Ph.D., Pioneer Health Crusader

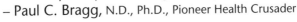

Super Oxygen Breathing for Super Living

When your body is fed with Live Foods and Super Oxygen, the joy of living will thrill you. Every day you bounce out of bed with a *glad to be alive* feeling, knowing there is meaning in life. You'll have fewer depressing thoughts, feelings, envy, jealousies, blue Mondays, hatreds, frustrations, fears, worries or morbid feelings!

With the stimulation of Super Oxygen, you are eager to meet life's problems. You meet them face to face and find solutions. You enjoy the effort of facing life's realities. You fully use the intelligence and common sense God gave you. Those people who know how to breathe deeply do not run away from life, but face it with courage and determination. The weakling, inevitably a shallow breather, takes the escape offered by alcohol, drugs and self-pity that leads to illness.

The Advantages of Super Power Breathing

• The most important of all physical acts is correct breathing. You can't be perfectly healthy if you don't breathe deeply. Super Power Breathing Exercises help you to practice the habit of correct breathing at all times.

• When you regularly breathe correctly, you add millions of health-giving, oxygen-carrying red blood cells to your bloodstream.

• When you fill your lungs with miracle-working oxygen, you cleanse your body of the toxic poisons that could do your body great damage.

• You will no longer crave artificial stimulants when sufficient oxygen is taken into your system. Oxygen is the only stimulant that has no harmful after-effects.

• When more oxygen gets into your bloodstream, you will feel super energized and will have greater vitality to better enjoy a longer, healthier life!

• Deep Super Power Breathing is now a part of all cures. Today, in the modern hospital, pure oxygen heals when every other method of healing has failed. Even broken bones heal more quickly when the blood is purified by doing daily Super Power Breathing Exercises.

Men do not die, they kill themselves. – Seneca, Roman Philosopher

More Advantages of Super Power Breathing

• Deep breathing is the great body normalizer. Oxygen is the invisible food for the body and helps with assimilation of the foods you have eaten. Super Power Breathing Exercises will also help people attain and maintain a more normal, healthy weight.

• <u>Many nervous diseases are due to oxygen starvation</u>. <u>Deep, diaphragmatic breathing tranquilizes jangled nerves and stimulates the brain to alertness and clear thinking to solve any of your life's problems</u>.

• If everyone practiced Super Power Breathing, there would be little need for eye, ear, nose and throat specialists. The oxygen filling these cavities destroys germs lodged there, and creates a healthier circulation.

• Many people suffer from poor circulation in various parts of the body. Because they don't get sufficient oxygen to produce a steady circulation of the blood into their extremities, they have cold hands, feet, noses and ears. The more oxygen you get into your body, the better your circulation and the warmer your hands and feet.

• People who get sufficient oxygen have better muscle tone. Their skin is healthier, firmer and more alive.

• Oxygen is Mother Nature's great beautifier. It gives the skin a radiant glow and the hair a lustrous sheen.

• People who inhale large amounts of oxygen are happier people. Deep breathing cleanses your body of psychological and physical poisons and gives you more joyful daily living and emotional well-being.

• Digestive ills are often helped by the internal massage of correct diaphragmatic action. When a Super Power Breath is taken, the digestive tract is exercised. *To help promote better digestion sip ½ tsp Bragg's Organic Apple Cider Vinegar before meals,* states Dr. Gabriel Cousens.

• Slow, deep breaths soothe and recharge the heart. Conversely, rapid, shallow breathing exhausts it through overwork and lack of sufficient oxygen for the blood.

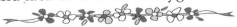

Bragg Super Power Breathing helps make the weak strong & athletes champions.
– Bob Anderson, world famous stretching coach (www.stretching.com)

More Advantages of Super Power Breathing

• Probably the last thing one would expect to be influenced by correct breathing is straightening of the teeth. Yet much corrective work done by the best American dental colleges on teeth and gums consists of deep diaphragmatic breathing. <u>Correct breathing helps normalizes the cavities of the nose, mouth and throat and exerts a gentle pressure upon the teeth</u>.

• Oxygen – the great invisible food, stimulant and purifier – builds our resistance to infections and strengthens our weak points. It's God's most vital aid in helping the body to heal itself and to stay healthy! Better an ounce of prevention, than a pound of cure!

Start now to breathe deeply and live fully!

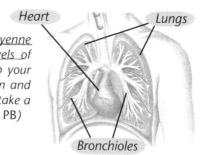

Heart Lungs

Bronchioles

A recent Japanese study has linked <u>cayenne (capsaicin) intake with improved levels of oxygen in the blood</u>. This helps keep your heart and cardiovascular system open and flowing and your brain more alert. (I take a 40,000 hu capsule of cayenne daily. – PB)

Studies prove that <u>free radicals are damaging substances that cause abnormal changes in cells that can lead to heart disease, cataracts, cancer and may be the cause of many of the effects attributed to premature ageing</u>. Antioxidants (found in fruits and vegetables) can trap and destroy these dangerous free radicals. Research shows that beta carotene – a powerful antioxidant found in carrots, cantaloupe and dark green vegetables – not only boosts the immune function, but is easily converted by the body to another important nutrient, vitamin A.

No man can violate Nature's Laws and escape her penalties. – Julian Johnson

---

The three greatest letters in the English alphabet are N-O-W.
There is no time like the present. Begin Now! – Sir Walter Scott, Scottish Poet

---

There are only two ways to live your life. One way is
as though nothing is a miracle. The other is as everything is a miracle!
– Albert Einstein

When we are sleeping or shallow breathing our lungs are getting only 10% of the oxygen that they can get. But when we deep breathe we are getting 80-90% of the oxygen we can get.

Chapter 19

Keep the Oxygen Coming For Life

Breathing is one of the most essential activities of life. We have already considered how, unlike with drinking or eating, we can live for only a very few short minutes without breathing. The work of bringing oxygen into the lungs and getting it into the bloodstream where it will be sent to nourish every cell of the body is the very basis of human life. It is for this reason that my father developed The Bragg Super Power Breathing. More than just a technique for better breathing, what we are describing to you in this book is a whole philosophy of breathing. By your mastering The Bragg Super Power Breathing you will maximize your lungs' capacity for oxygenating your body and your capacity for making use of this vital nourishment, the invisible staff of life.

But even The Bragg Super Power Breathing can't guarantee that you will always be getting the oxygen you need. Emergency rescue personnel, medics, lifeguards and others around the country and around the world can attest to this: even the healthiest, fittest, most vital of people can suddenly and unexpectedly be threatened with oxygen starvation. Unlike the slow suffocation most people suffer because of bad breathing habits, sudden suffocation refers to dangers of choking, drowning, asthma attacks and other events that can deprive a person of needed, life-giving oxygen. (See pages 130-131)

The Bragg Healthy Lifestyle, along with Super Power Breathing (SPB), can go a long way in helping asthmatics overcome dangerous effects of their breathing condition, though the onset of an asthmatic attack still threatens the SPB breather with oxygen deprivation. Likewise, the choking or drowning victim who is a SPB will suffocate just the same, unless the object or water is removed.

The Lord gives strength to those who are weary. – Isaiah 40:29

Perfect health is above gold; a sound body before riches. – Solomon

The Heimlich Maneuver Jumpstarts the Lungs

My father and I want to do all we can to ensure that all people are able to get all the oxygen they need. We have even included how to get the asthma or choking and drowning accident victims breathing again, page 130.

Many of you are familiar with the famous Heimlich Maneuver* as a technique for saving choking victims. Since 1974, this procedure has saved more than 50,000 lives just in the United States. This maneuver, developed by Dr. Henry J. Heimlich, is performed by pressing upward on the diaphragm. This compresses the lungs, causing a flow of air that helps push the choking object out that is blocking the airway. Recent evidence and research has suggested the Heimlich Maneuver is effective in restoring breathing in more emergency situations than just choking. Our friends Dr. Heimlich along with his wife Jane Murray Heimlich is, *the daughter of famous Arthur and Katherine Murray who taught America to dance,* have dedicated their lives to educating the world about the life-saving Heimlich Maneuver. www.heimlichinstitute.org

Heimlich Helps Save Drowning Victims

In more than 90% of drowning cases, the victim's lungs fill with fluid. In this situation, it is imperative that the fluid be expelled quickly - because after four or five minutes the likelihood of brain damage increases. Just getting someone out of the water has not changed their condition - if they still have fluid in their lungs their condition is the same as if they were still under water. In all the studies on drowning since 1933, none showed that mouth-to-mouth resuscitation saved drowning victims without first draining water from their lungs. After all, air cannot get into water-filled lungs!

The Heimlich Maneuver expels water from lungs of drowning victims in six to nine seconds – with two to four Heimlich applications. And unlike CPR, when applied correctly, Heimlich is safe and easily mastered by a person new to the procedure. Option: hold drown victim upside down to drain water out, then apply CPR if needed.

---

* Heimlich Institute, 311 Straight St., Cincinnati, OH 45219 • (513) 559-2391or 419-7062
Call your local radio stations and suggest Dr.Heimlich is a perfect talk show guest.

CPR unfortunately often causes rib fractures, lung punctures, internal bleeding and injuries of all sorts. In one study of 323 people who died after receiving CPR, 17% of the people likely died of injuries caused by CPR! Adding to the danger of using CPR in asphyxiation situations, another study finds that in 86% of the cases, a drowning (or choking) victim vomits after resuscitation by CPR. Vomiting can cause airway blockage and death if not cleared. (It happened to a friend. Most ambulances carry airway tubes for this, but his didn't.) In contrast, less than 3% of cases vomited after safer Heimlich Maneuver.

Take the advice of the National Pool and Water Park Association and learn the Heimlich Maneuver - the resuscitation technique they recommend as the first step in treating drowning victims. Results prove it works!

Heimlich Maneuver Helps Combat Asthma

Today over 18 million Americans suffer from asthma, 6 million are under the age of 18. Asthma accounts for 1.8 million emergency room visits and 10 million office doctor visits a year. It's one of the great maladies of our modern, polluted, poisoned age. Five thousand Americans die from asthma every year, 14 every day. An asthma attack occurs when muscles surrounding the airway contract, narrowing air passages that, in the case of asthmatics, are chronically swollen and inflamed. During an attack, mucus fills airway like a plug. When the victim breathes in, the air slides around the mucus obstructions. When the victim tries to exhale, the mucus plugs the airway, stopping flow of air out of lungs. This situation often makes the use of asthma inhalers ineffective in relieving an attack. (See page 131, it's getting good results.)

Even in emergency rooms with all that modern technology and pharmacological medicine they offer, more people are dying of asthma. Last year, 22 children died of asthma attacks in one New York City emergency room alone. There is hope for the victims of asthma attacks. Our friends Dr. Henry Heimlich and his author wife Jane Murray Heimlich are real crusaders doing their best to help people worldwide. They are saving lives!

I've seen partially paralyzed, stroke and accident patients, half carried into a hyperbaric oxygen chamber, and walk out after their first treatment! – Dr. Edgar End

First Aid for Choking & Drowning Victims
The Heimlich Maneuver

With the VICTIM STANDING or SITTING

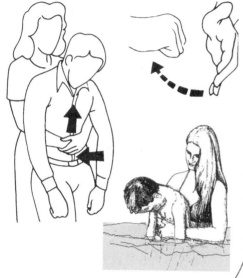

1. Stand behind the victim and wrap your arms firmly around their upper waist.

2. Place the thumb side of your fist strongly against the victim's abdomen, slightly just above the navel and below the rib cage.

3. Grasp your fist with your other hand and press fist into the upper abdomen with a **quick upward thrust. Repeat often as necessary.**

4. If the victim is sitting, stand behind the victim's chair and perform maneuver in the same manner. Never slap victims' back.

5. After food, etc. is removed, have the victim seen by a doctor immediately.

Note: If you start to choke when alone and help is not available, an attempt should be made to self-administer this Heimlich Maneuver.

When the VICTIM HAS COLLAPSED and CANNOT BE LIFTED:

1. Lay the victim on their back.

2. Face the victim and kneel astride victims hips and thighs.

3. With one hand on top of another, place heel of bottom hand on upper abdomen slightly above navel and below the rib cage.

4. Press into the victim's upper abdomen with a QUICK UPWARD THRUST. Don't squeeze ribcage. Repeat as often as necessary.

5. Should victim vomit, quickly place them on their side and wipe out any vomit from mouth to prevent blocking of throat and aspiration *(drawing vomit into throat). (Ambulances have suction & airway tubes.)*

6. After food, water, etc. is removed, give CPR if needed and it's best to have the victim seen by a doctor immediatly.

Everyone should know the versatile Heimlich Maneuver for it's a life-saver!
– Visit Dr. Heimlich's website: www.heimlichinstitute.org

Heimlich Maneuver Stops Asthma Attacks

A growing body of cases documents the effectiveness of the Heimlich Maneuver in stopping asthma attacks. As Dr. Heimlich explains, *"We started receiving calls from people who had suffered severe, almost deadly asthma attacks. The people who were with them didn't have any idea what to do. And off the top of their heads, they used the Heimlich Maneuver. They just tried it,"* he says, *"and immediately, a miracle happened, the asthma attack stopped."*

When the diaphragm of an asthma attack victim is pushed up with the Heimlich Maneuver (whether self-applied or not), the lungs become compressed. When this happens, the trapped air is forcibly expelled and the air flow carries away the mucus plugs that started the attack. After the maneuver, the airway is cleared and the asthma attack ends. When performed on asthmatics, the Heimlich Maneuver need only be done very gently because you are expelling mucus and trapped air – not a stuck, solid object, food, etc. or lungs full of water.

There is also good evidence that the versatile Heimlich Maneuver can prevent an asthma attack from occurring. Studies show that applying the procedure on a regular basis keeps the lungs free of the mucus that can plug up the airway and bring on an asthma attack.

I've seen asthma disappear completely in response to major shifts in diet and lifestyles, such as eliminating sugar, milk and switching to a healthier, vegetarian diet. – Dr. Andrew Weil, *Self Healing Newsletter.*

Stay away from milk – it's a killer! – Dr. Virgil Hulse, M.D.
Author of: *Mad Cows and Milk Gate* – available (541) 482-2048 Also Amazon.com

---

Breathe deeply and allow yourself to be filled with life energizing oxygen for a vital life filled with health, energy, laughter, peace and love.
– Patricia Bragg, N.D., Ph.D., Health Crusader.

Hollywood actress Cloris Leachman, now a healthy vegetarian who sparkles with health, says, "Fasting is simply wonderful. It's my solution to many problems. It is a miracle cure for sure. . . it cured my asthma."

A strong body makes a strong mind. – Thomas Jefferson

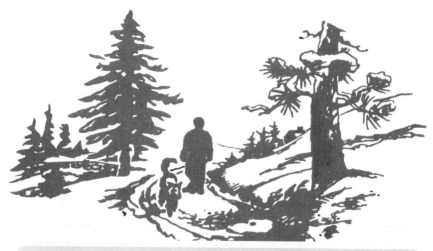

Mind Food for Wise Healthy Living

One of the most tragic things about human nature is that all of us tend to put off living. We are dreaming of some magical rose garden over the horizon – instead of enjoying the roses that are blooming outside our windows today.
– Dale Carnegie

As the tide of chemicals born in the Industrial Age has arisen to engulf our environment, a drastic change has come about in the nature of the most serious public health problem. For the first time in the history of the world, every human being is now subject to contact with dangerous chemicals, from the moment of conception until death. – Rachel Carson, *Silent Spring*, 1962 classic

Old age is not a time of life. It's a condition of the body. It's not time that ages the body, it's abuse that does! – Herbert Shelton

It's supposed to be a professional secret, but I'll tell you anyway. We doctors do nothing. We only help and encourage the doctor within. – Albert Schweitzer

Happiness is the meaning and the purpose of life, the whole aim of human existence. – Aristotle

We all grow healthier in nature, gentle sunshine and love!

Nothing in all creation is so like God as stillness. – Meister Eckhart

Man's body was created according to the laws of physics and chemistry, which are the Creator's own laws. They never vary. His law is written upon every nerve, every muscle, every faculty, which has been entrusted to us. – Henry W. Vollmer, M.D.

Kindness should be a frame of mind in which we are alert to every chance: to do, to give, to share and to cheer. – Patricia Bragg

Smile at yourself, smile at your wife, smile at your husband, smile at your children, smile at each other – it doesn't matter who it is – and that will help you grow in greater love for each other. – Mother Teresa

Chapter 20

Doctor Fresh Air

Dr. Fresh Air is a Super Health Specialist and his greatest prescription is *The Breath of God's Pure Fresh Air, the Invisible Staff of Life.*

The first thing we do when we are born is to take a long, deep breath and the final thing we do is take a last gasp before we stop breathing. Between birth and death our life is completely maintained by our breathing.

Dr. Fresh Air wants you to have a long, healthy life. Practice these Bragg Super Power Breathing exercises and remain conscious that with every breath you take you are bringing into your body precious life-giving oxygen.

People who fail to obey the doctor's orders about getting plenty of fresh air day and night invite extremely severe complications. Let us examine the function of breathing. It is invisible food – the only food that we absolutely cannot live without. If we are deprived of air for over 5 to 7 minutes, death will take us. We are miracle breathing machines. Nurture, protect and honor your life.

Air supplies us with life-giving oxygen, which is critical for every cell in our bodies. Oxygen is carried by the blood to the lungs where a great miracle takes place: the exchange of life-giving oxygen for deadly carbon dioxide. We create deadly toxins in the process of living that CO_2 carries out of our bodies. These are collected by our blood, brought to our lungs and expelled as the new life-giving oxygen enters our bloodstream. During the process of metabolism, the building up and tearing down of the cells of the body, and in the very process of living, carbon dioxide poison is constantly burned up.

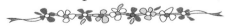

You are what you breathe, eat, drink, think, say and do! – Patricia Bragg, N.D., Ph.D..

Look at your own life. Has it become overly complex? Have you found yourself burdened by too many possessions or responsibilities? Take a slow, deep breath and ask yourself: "What steps can I take to reduce the clutter so that I may live life simply and joyously?" – Douglas Bloch

We are Miracle Air Breathing Machines

When a person does not get enough fresh air – or is a shallow breather – and their intake of oxygen does not equal the output of carbon dioxide, then this poison can build up in the body. This could result in serious physical problems because the retained carbon dioxide can be concentrated in other parts of the body and could cause intense physical problems and suffering.

WEAKEN NERVE

Enervation is the lack of nerve energy that lowers the Vital Force so much that the lungs cannot pump in enough air to flush carbon dioxide out of the body. Now you see how important it is to breathe fresh air deeply and do your Super Power Breathing exercises every day!

We are air-pressure machines and oxygen purifies our bodies. It's one of the greatest detoxifiers of the human body. We live at the bottom of an atmospheric ocean approximately 70 miles deep. This air pressure is 14 pounds per square inch. Between the inhalation and the exhalation of a breath, a vacuum is formed. As long as we continue to have this rhythmical intake of oxygen and outflow of carbon dioxide, we will live. We know that we can go without food for 30 days or more and still survive, but we can only go without air for a few minutes. Air is one of the most important energizers of the human body. The more deeply you breathe, the better your chances for extending your years on Earth.

For over 70 years, my father researched long-lived people and found one common factor among them: they are deep breathers! The deeper – and therefore fewer – breaths a person takes in one minute, the longer that person lives. Rapid breathers are short-lived. This holds true in the animal world, too. Rabbits, guinea pigs and all kinds of rodents are rapid breathers, taking many breaths every minute. They are among the shortest-lived creatures on the face of Earth. For years we have made it a practice to take long, slow, deep breaths when we first get up in the morning. During the day, we also try to take periods where we breathe long, deeper full breaths. Try this now – it makes you feel wonderfully alive!

Indian Holy Men Practice Slow, Deep Breathing and Meditation

On my father's expeditions into India, he found holy men in secluded retreats who devoted their lives to building physically powerful bodies as instruments for high spiritual advancement. They spent many hours daily in the practice of rhythmic, relaxed, long, slow, deep breathing. These holy men of India were utterly fantastic physically. The deep breathing of fresh air kept their skin and muscle-tone ageless. Dad met a holy man in the foothills of the Himalaya Mountains who told him that he was 126 years old. This man's whole life was spent in getting closer to God. He is the one who taught my father the system which we expanded upon and now teach all over the world as *Bragg Super Power Breathing.*

This holy man had perfect vision and he had a beautiful head of hair. He had all his teeth and the endurance and stamina of an athlete. He also spoke five languages fluently. He was one of the most amazing men my father ever met! When asked to what he owed his great strength and mentality, he answered, *"I have made a lifelong practice of faithfully doing my deep breathing and deep, slow breathing meditations daily."* (This is their prayer.)

My father does not like to guess the age of any person, but while he was on this trip to India he met a woman whose age he guessed to be about 50. He was amazed when she told him she was 86! She was a beautiful woman with virtually no sign of deterioration. He was impressed and asked her the secret of her beauty and her agelessness. Again he got the same answer he did from the holy man, this beautiful woman was conscious of the importance of deep, slow breathing and prayer.

Man's days shall be to 120 years. – Genesis 6:3

Perfect health is above gold; a sound body before riches. – Solomon

Slow, deep breathing and relaxation techniques are important health benefits to the entire body's system. Such techniques as sitting quietly, ignoring distracting thoughts, meditating and praying can bring down blood pressure and have no side effects. – Harvard Health Letter

135

Super Power Deep Breathing:
Secret of Endurance, Stamina & Longevity

No doubt you have noticed rosy-cheeked children playing – running and jumping rope, roller-skating and bicycling. They inhale large amounts of oxygen while doing these activities, and that is what we must keep in mind. We must keep active! We must exercise and take long, brisk walks and cultivate deep breathing. When people live sedentary, uncreative lives and no longer get vigorous exercise, they are harming themselves and shortening their lives.

We had a long-time friend named Amos Stagg who was a famous California football and athletic coach. He lived over 100 active, happy years. We asked him his secret of long life at his 100th birthday party. His answer was, *"I have the greater part of my life indulged in running and other vigorous exercise that forced large amounts of oxygen into my body and along with working with athletes, has kept me youthful and interested in staying alive."*

Dad had a friend in New York, James Hocking, who was one of the greatest long-distance walking champions this country has ever had. We asked him on his 100th birthday the secret of his long, active life, super healthy life. His answer was, *"I have always walked vigorously and breathed deeply."* Oxygen is a cleansing detoxifier like fasting and it helps remove toxins from the body.

We both practice deep breathing and believe people should expose their bodies to free currents of moving air. Air baths are important for good health. Whenever possible do sleep with your windows wide open with cross ventilated air moving across your body. We sleep better and have a deeper night's rest if we wear light sleeping garments of cotton or silk – or nothing at all. You will be warm under the covers. But if you sleep with heavy blankets and nightwear, you smother your skin's vital oxygen supply and increase your chance of illness.

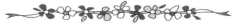

Control your emotions by learning to breathe through them.

Our breathing is a very convenient process to support the ongoing awareness in our daily lives. – Jon Kabat-Zinn, Ph.D.

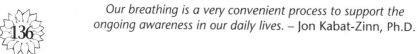

Healthy Walking Helps Solve Problems

You will find that you can solve most of your problems on a brisk one to three mile hike. Whenever we have a problem to solve, we always take a long brisk walk in the fresh air and even if raining (Conrad Hilton walked rain or shine). By the time we finish our walk, we usually find a solution! We believe that everyone should make a practice of taking brisk short walks (arms swinging) hour after their evening meal – even if it is up and down their driveway. Today people have become sitters. They sit at their workplace, movies, concerts and while watching sports and TV at home. They are starved for more oxygen, exercise and circulation!

You must compensate for the hours you spend sitting down, because it inhibits your circulation and natural, healthy breathing. If your work and lifestyle require a lot of sitting, you should compensate for it with outdoor brisk walking and more vigorous physical activities.

When you cannot get the carbon dioxide out of your body, you develop aches, pains and become prone to premature ageing. This is due to lack of physical activity and sufficient oxygen. On city streets, you can see pale, ghostly people, unhealthy and exhausted – mostly as a result of oxygen-starvation and poor lifestyle choices.

It's critical to fast, because it enables you to clean out some of this concentrated, stored-up carbon dioxide that failed to leave your body by deep breathing. When you are fasting, enjoy walking – even if it is a short walk. Make it a regular part of your life to be an active person. This doesn't mean house walks. It means getting out in the fresh air and hiking, biking, running, swimming or dancing, etc. You must not allow any carbon dioxide to build up in your body – it will bring health problems!

Make it a point every day of your life to breathe deeply during a vigorous brisk walk or some other aerobic exercise. Take long, slow, deep breaths every time you think of it. Soon your slow, deep breathing becomes a normal habit. When you combine deep breathing with fasting and living The Bragg Healthy Lifestyle, you are building more health, energy and vitality and you will live longer. Remind yourself every day that Doctor Fresh Air is your very important constant friend!

HEALTHY HEART HABITS FOR A LONG, VITAL LIFE

Remember, *organic live foods make live people. You are what you eat, drink, breathe, think, say and do.* So eat a low-fat, low-sugar, high-fiber diet of organic whole grains, sprouts, fresh salads, organic greens, vegetables, fruits, raw seeds, nuts, fresh juices and chemical-free, purified or distilled water.

Earn your food with daily exercise; for regular exercise, brisk walking, aerobics, etc. improves health, stamina, go-power, flexibility and endurance and helps open the cardiovascular system. Only 45 minutes a day truly can do miracles for your heart, arteries, mind, nerves, soul and body! You become revitalized with new zest for living to accomplish your life goals!

We are made of tubes. To help keep them open, clean and to maintain good elimination, add 1 Tbsp of psyllium husk powder daily – hour after dinner – to juices, herbal teas and even the Bragg Vinegar Drink. Another way to guard against clogged tubes daily is add 1 to 2 Tbsps soy lecithin granules (*fat emulsifier-melts like butter*) over potatoes, veggies, soups and to juices, etc. Also take one cayenne capsule (40,000 HU) daily with a meal. Take 50 to 100 mgs regular-released niacin (B-3) with one meal daily to help cleanse and open the cardiovascular system, also improves memory. Skin flushing may occur; don't worry about this as it shows it's working! After cholesterol level reaches 180 then only take niacin twice weekly. Also studies show ½ tsp cinnamon powder is natures *statin* with no side effects.

The heart needs healthy balanced nutrients, so take natural multi-vitamin-mineral food supplements & extra heart helpers – mixed vitamin E, C, CoQ10, magnesium orotate, Omega-3, MSM, selenium, zinc, beta carotene & amino acids L-Carnitine, L-Taurine, L-Lysine & Proline. Folic acid, CoQ10, B6 & B12 helps keep homocysteine & CRP levels low. Hawthorn Berry extract brings relief for palpitations, arrhythmia, senile hearts and coronary disease. Take bromelain (from pineapple) and a multi-digestive enzyme with meals – aids and improves digestion, assimilation and elimination.

For sleep problems try melatonin, 5-HTP tryptophan (an amino acid), calcium, magnesium, valerian in caps, extract or tea, Bragg vinegar drink, chamomile or sleepytime herbal tea. For arthritis, osteoarthritis, pain/stiffness, try aloe gel or aloe juice, glucosamine, chondroitin & MSM combo (caps, liquid & rollon) helps heal & regenerate. Also capsaicin & DMSO lotion helps heal.

Use amazing antioxidants – natural vitamin mixed E, C, Quercetin, grapeseed and grapefruit extract, CoQ10, selenium, SOD, etc. They improve immune system and help flush out dangerous free radicals that cause havoc with cardiovascular pipes and health. Research shows that antioxidants and enzymes promote longevity, slows ageing, fights toxins and cancer and helps prevent disease, cancer, cataracts, jet lag and exhaustion.

Recommended Blood Chemistry Values

- **Homocysteine:** 6 - 8 mcm/L • **CRP (C-reactive protein high sensitivity):** lower than 1 mg/L low risk, 1-3 mg/L average risk, over 3 mg/L high risk
- **Total Cholesterol: Adults,** 180 mg/dl or less; 150 mg/dl is optimal **Children,** 140 mg/dl or less
- **HDL Cholesterol:** Men, 50 mg/dl or more; Women, 65 mg/dl or more
- **HDL Cholesterol Ratio:** 3.2 or less • **Triglycerides:** 100 mg/dl or less
- **LDL Cholesterol:** 100 mg/dl or less is optimal • **Glucose:** 80-100 mg/dl

Chapter 21

Doctor Rest –
The Recharger of Life

Doctor Rest is another specialist always at your command to help you achieve Supreme Vitality. We believe the word *rest* is the most misunderstood word in the English language. Some people's idea of resting is to sit down and drink a cup of a strong stimulant such as coffee, black tea or caffeinated soft drinks. This is typified by the *coffee break*. To us, rest means repose, freedom from activity and quiet tranquility. It means peace of mind and spirit. It means to rest without anxiety or worry. And it means to refresh oneself. Your rest should renew your whole nervous system and your entire body.

QUITENESS, CALM

When you're resting, you shouldn't sit with one leg crossed over the other because this position puts a heavy burden on the artery which supplies the feet with blood and also cuts off nerve energy. If you sit with your legs crossed you are not resting, but giving your heart an extra load of work to do! When you sit down, it's best to keep both feet on the floor or a footstool.

To rest means to allow free circulation (no restrictions) of blood throughout the body, which is important for health. Are your shoes too tight? Your collar? Your hat? Your stockings? Your belt, watch or *undergarments? If yes, then you're not resting when you sit or lie down!

Why do we rest? Often people say, *"I need to rest!"* Yet when they sit down intending to rest, they nervously drum their fingers on a table or desk, quiver or shake their legs or they squirm and move about restlessly.

The art of resting is something that must be acquired and concentrated upon. The best rest can only be secured when your body is relaxed and freed from restrictive clothing. Your clothes should be comfortably loose.

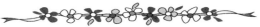

* Read *Dressed To Kill,* by Sydney Singer, on breast cancer and bra studies.
(I've never worn a bra, only a loose chemise. – Patricia Bragg)
Visit ISCDPress.com – Singer Books available amazon.com

Enjoy Rest & Naps – It's Not a Crime to Relax!

One good way to rest is to lie down on a firm bed, unclothed or wearing as few, loose clothes as possible. Another good way to rest is to sunbathe – pg 152 -155. There is nothing that will relax the muscles and nerves like the gentle, soothing early morning or late afternoon sun rays. In order to rest and nap, you must learn to clear your mind of all anxiety, worries and emotional problems. When the muscles and nerves are relaxed, the heart action slows – especially when you take long, slow, deep breaths. This will help promote a deeper relaxation and more total rest for more total health!

Another good form of resting is a short nap. When you take a nap, command your muscles to become completely relaxed. Your conscious and subconscious mind controls the muscles and the nerves, so you must be in complete command of your body when you rest. Jesus said to His Disciples, when worn and weary, "Come ye and rest a while." The Master did not lead them into the busy streets of Jerusalem where there was noise and clatter. He didn't even take them into the church. He took them into the quiet wide open spaces of nature, under the blue sky. There they could rebuild, relax and revive every organ of their exhausted bodies and also revitalize, refresh and invigorate their weary minds. The greatest place to rest, relax and renew your body's Vital Force is under the blue sky, in the clean, fresh air. On hot summer days, enjoy the cool shade of trees.

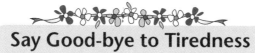

Say Good-bye to Tiredness

- Sit down and kick off your shoes. Let tiredness go and now relax!
- Now start breathing in easily and deeply. Breathe out tiredness.
  Breathe deeply in a feeling of peace and relaxation.
- Curl your toes down tight, now relax toes and feet. Repeat exercise:
  Now tighten, then relax fingers and slowly do your arms, legs, etc.
- Breathe out slowly all the pressures and tiredness of the day.
  Then breathe in refreshing joy, health, love and peace.
     Now it's time to stand up and stretch. . .
- Stand, stretch up. Swing arms up and do wide circles, then reverse circles.
- Now stretch your body, arms and legs – sideways, up and down, etc.

Breathe deeply in life and breathe out stress, tension, etc.

Sleep – The Miracle Recharger

Sleep is the greatest revitalizer we have, but few people get a long, peaceful and refreshing night's sleep. Most people habitually use stimulants like tobacco, drugs, coffee, tea and other caffeinated drinks which batter tired nerves. People who use these toxic stimulants never have complete rest and relaxation because their nerves are always in an excited condition.

Most people do not earn their rest. Rest must be earned with physical and mental activity, because they go hand in hand. So many people complain what poor sleepers they are – that they toss and turn throughout the night. For an extra relaxer before bedtime try our Bragg Apple Cider Health Drink hot or cold (It's delicious; see recipe on page 116), (More sleep info page 136).

Today, millions of people take some type of drug to induce sleep, but this is not true sleep. No one gets restful sleep with any sleeping tablets. You may drug yourself into unconsciousness, but that very drug will deprive you of a normal, restful, healthy and satisfying sleep.

Healthy Lifestyle Promotes Sound Sleep

Your nerves are continually irritated when you do not eliminate the toxins from your body. How is it possible to get a good night's rest with irritated nerves? When we live our Healthy Lifestyle, exercise, breathe deeply and perform our weekly 24 hour fast, we enjoy sound sleep. We have discovered that when our students discard their stimulants and begin a regular fasting program, they too enjoy a more restful, deep sleep.

You will notice as you purify your body that you will be able to relax more readily. You will be able to enjoy naps and you will reap the benefits of a long, restful, night's sleep. Rest is important! The Bible tells us that God appointed one day of rest every week for man. In this wise law, we have ample support for our contention that frequent changes of activity is an important factor in maintaining Super Health. To complement our busy days, we require and enjoy a variety of fun recreational activities. This old adage is true and wise advice to follow: *All work and no play does make Jack and Jill dull and tired.*

Life is to be Savored and Enjoyed – Not Hectic

Today we live in a hectic, competitive environment, which the business world calls the *rat race*. During these stressful times filled with political and emotional unrest, we build up tremendous pressures, tensions and strains. This is why people turn to tobacco, drugs, coffee, alcohol and other harmful substances – to try to escape the stress.

There is not only competition in the business world, but in the social realm as well, as people strive to maintain their *status*. People are always trying to impress one another and trying to create a certain *image*. Often they create a false image and it takes energy to portray this falseness! There is tremendous pressure on women who believe their worth is being dependent on their appearance. So they spend hours having their hair and nails colored, constantly trying to keep up with the latest fashions, struggling to have a different – *perfect* – body. All of this calls for energy. Our modern civilization drives and pushes us, robbing us of our natural, peaceful state.

It's no wonder we have created millions of alcoholics and drug addicts. Why have people completely forgotten that life is meant to be lived and enjoyed? Too few individuals these days enjoy leisure living. Life is one big rush! Where and why is everyone rushing these days? It's best to slow down, relax - get healthy and happy!

To be able to relax, rest and sleep you must program your day so you have balanced time for work, rest, recreation, exercise and a good night's sleep. Also, you can't get a good sleep if you overload your stomach. You will enjoy better sleep if you earn it with daily exercise, brisk walking, gardening, etc. We have love and concern for you and love being your health teachers and friends to inspire you to live The Bragg Healthy Lifestyle. Please nourish your body with healthy natural foods, pure distilled water, lots of fresh air, exercise and deep breathing exercises.

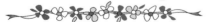

People who say it can't be done shouldn't interrupt those who are doing it!

I have the wisdom of my years and the youthfulness of The Bragg Healthy Lifestyle and I never act or feel my calendar years! I feel ageless! So why shouldn't you? Start living this Bragg Healthy Way today! – Patricia Bragg

Love Mother Nature, God and Yourself Daily

Enjoy a balanced program of exercise and repose and let Mother Nature and God do the rest! Treat yourself as you deserve and the results will astound you! We, the *Back to Nature People*, have been ridiculed for years as faddists and extremists. Now our healthy lifestyle is in demand! The popular press prints stories daily confirming what we have always known! We believe in Mother Nature and God and want to spread their health, love, joy, peace and happiness worldwide. Read *3 John 2* and *Genesis 6:3*.

We recommend that you return to a more natural way of living in food, clothing, rest and in simplicity of living habits. Strive for harmony with Mother Nature and God. Live as Mother Nature wants. Realize that she loves you and you are part of her family. Put yourself in her hands and let her inner wisdom guide you. Mother Nature is eager to inspire and guide you so she can help you perfect your human machine. She can help cleanse, heal and improve your body if you work with her by living a healthier life. Follow the Bragg Healthy Lifestyle.

When possible, leave the smog-filled, air-polluted cities for the country. In the quiet beauty of meadow and hill, you will rekindle your youth. For success: plan, plot and follow through with a strong belief you will become healthier and more youthful! If you live in a city, make it a point to go enjoy your parks, the country or the seashore where you can find clean air, relaxation, in a peaceful natural setting for beautiful, recharging retreat time for your body, mind and soul.

Breathing deeply, fully and completely energizes the body, calms the nerves, fills you with peace and helps keep you youthful. – Paul C. Bragg, N.D., Ph.D.

Romance with God and Mother Nature never grows stale, they walk with you and talk with you and their wisdom is thrilling! – Patricia Bragg, N.D., Ph.D.

Aromatherapy – A Healer For Centuries

You will enjoy a wonderful experience and enhance your health. Aromatherapy has the power to work miracles, to uplift and heal. Essential oils can help improve physical and emotional health. Treat yourself to the delights and fragrances of essential oils. Smelling roses, flowers and fruit blossoms is also recharging.

Tips for Healthy, Peaceful Living

• Regard your body as a wonderful miracle machine, 100% under your care and control. Become your own health captain and guardian of your habits of living so that you may be well balanced for a lifetime of health.

• Demand of yourself a higher standard of healthy lifestyle habits. Recognize that every machine must have rest periods. You can't receive higher, super health unless your body gets its rest periods to develop new found vitality and boundless energy. Without sufficient rest, health problems build up when your vital nerve force is depleted. The majority of Americans are stressed-out and unhealthy. Read the Bragg *Nerve Force* book for more info about building powerful, healthy, peaceful nerves.

• You will become wiser and more mature when you draw closer to and become more intimate with God and Mother Nature. Stop seeking overstimulation and thrills; instead, seek a simple, "back to nature" peaceful life. Be faithful and you will have a healthy, long and active life God and Mother Nature intended for you to enjoy.

Man's days shall be 120 years. – Genesis 6:3

• With a clear eye and confidence, put yourself in their loving care. They will run your human machine, heal your hurts, comfort you in sickness and adversity. Then, when you have lived a long life of usefulness and happiness, you will be called home (Psalms 23). Make them your life partner, and when you are resting, relaxing, and building new energy, they will always be there for you. So be a child of God and Mother Nature – don't look for sophisticated thrills! Find your fun and diversion in relaxation and other pursuits that are simple as 1, 2, 3. Your rewards will be many: renewed health, calm spirit and a new awareness of the perfect beauties that Mother Nature and our Creator have generously bestowed on us!

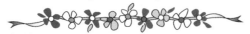

You are encircled by the arms of the mystery of God. – Hildegard of Bingen

During your weekly 24 hour fast try to avoid criticizing anyone or anything! Fill yourself only with loving, positive thoughts, not only on your fasting and cleansing days, but everyday! Before you speak put your words to this test! Is it good? Is it kind? Is it necessary? If not, don't speak! – Patricia Bragg

Chapter 22

Doctor Exercise
Activity is Life, Stagnation is Death

Doctor Exercise makes this assertion . . .*To be lazy is to rust and rust means decay and destruction.* If we don't use our muscles, they loose their tone and life! To keep muscles firm, strong and youthful, they must be continually used! Activity is the Law of Health and Life! Action is the Law of Well-Being! All the body's vital organs have specific functions that depend upon health and strength. Exercise helps normalize weight, blood pressure, blood sugar and cholesterol and fat levels.

When we exercise, we increase physical strength, stamina, suppleness and good circulation. Daily exercise improves digestion, elimination and strengthens the muscles, especially the heart. If we are lazy and don't use our 640 muscles, our circulation, muscles and health all suffer from lack of exercise. The unused muscles become flabby, weak, unhealthy and unable to enjoy active exercise and a normal healthy, vigorous life.

People who exercise regularly have better skin tone. When we exercise, we bring on healthy perspiration from our body's 96 million pores. (Health Clubs have steam and sauna rooms that open your pores.) Skin is the body's largest eliminative organ (often called your third kidney). If someone gilded your body, clogging all your pores, you would die within minutes.

When you are exercising and perspiring freely, impurities and toxic poisons are expelled. This allows the skin to perform its natural function of eliminating these poisons. If you don't exercise daily to the point of perspiration, the work that the pores should be doing throws a double burden on the other eliminative organs and then physical trouble can occur. Vigorous exercise helps to normalize blood pressure and helps create a healthier pulse. Vigorous exercise acts as an anticoagulant, which means that it helps keep the blood from forming the clots which can cause a heart attack or stroke. Remember, daily brisk walking works miracles.

Exercise Promotes Healthy Elimination

Every creature and human eliminates internal waste by means of muscular action. Inside your intestinal tract, there are three muscular layers which undergo a precise rhythmic, *wavelike-squeeze-push* called peristalsis. If you allow the internal and external abdominal muscles (important for elimination) to become inactive, flabby and fat instead of muscular, they lose their power to contract normally. The results: intestinal clogging which can cause constipation and even diarrhea at times.

What happens when stomach muscles become weak and infiltrated with fat? They often refuse to work regularly. Then intestinal waste that should have been eliminated piles up. Fecal and toxic waste build-ups cause ill health. This sluggish inactivity can cause many diseases.

Fasting and a healthy lifestyle are your friends in your pursuit of youthfulness, health and symmetry. When it comes to fighting fat – diet and fasting come first. But when it comes to keeping fit, exercise matters most. However, they all help each other; by taking exercise you may be more generous with your diet. The human machine should work well and enjoy the highest peak of efficiency. All machines improve with intelligent use, and nothing betrays its weak spots as much as inactivity, lack of maintenance and inadequate, low-energy fuel! For example: your car needs routine maintenance including gas, oil changes, tune-ups, etc.

Enjoy Brisk Walks for Healthy Long Life

We recommend most all forms of exercise, but feel daily brisk walking with arms swinging, is the best all-around exercise. Walking moves most of the body. Grasp the small of your back as you walk and feel how your entire frame responds to every stride and how the muscles work rhythmically. Walking promotes harmony of all the body's coordinating muscles. Your daily walk promotes healthier blood circulation, elimination, deeper breathing and helps normalize blood pressure even diabetes and cholesterol.

The Bragg Healthy Lifestyle and brisk walking (3X daily) for 20 minutes after meals, helped me eliminate my diabetes! My whole body, circulation, feet, eyes have improved. Thank you, may God continue to bless your Crusade. – John Risk, Santee, CA

Walking is the King of Exercise

Walking does not need to be done consciously. No heel and toe business. No getting there within a certain time limit. Let walking be as it is: the most functional of exercises. Carry yourself well. Walk naturally with your head high and chest up. You will feel physically elated and you will carry yourself proudly, straight and erect – yet relaxed and with an easy, smooth arm-swing.

Vow to become a wonderful walker and make the day's walk a fixed item in your health program all the year round and in any kind of weather. Go at your own pace with your spirit free. If the outer world of Mother Nature fails to interest you, turn to the inner world of the mind. (Science now says adults can grow new brain cells.)

In our opinion walking is better than golf. Life has so much to teach us that it's a time-waster trying to get a ball into a hole in a stroke less than another person. Unfortunately most golfers now use electric golf carts which eliminates the best part of golf – walking!

Gardening is a marvelous form of exercise. It gives you exercise in the open air to help keep you more flexible. But you can gain weight even if you garden because there is too little movement. Therefore, we prefer walking, even though both are good for you. Achieve your goals by applying your energy productively in your organic vegetable and flower gardens, then take the kink out of your back with a healthy brisk walk and stretching. Personally, we enjoy combining these: swimming, tennis, biking, calisthenics, hiking and brisk walking. We also love garden exercise. We have a variety of organic fruit trees, vegetables, herbs and flower gardens with over 350 perfume roses. My father said "Roses are God's Autograph".

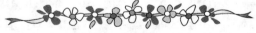

If you don't use it, you lose it – it's true in mind, body and spirit.

Now learn what great benefits a temperate diet will bring with it. In the first place, you will enjoy good health. – Horace, 65 B.C.

Our best preparation for tomorrow is the proper use of today.

The Importance of Abdominal Exercises

The most important exercises stimulate all of the muscles of the human trunk from the hips to the armpits. These are the binding muscles which hold all of the vital organs in place. In developing your torso muscles, you are also developing the vital muscles. As your back, waist, chest and abdomen increase in soundness and elasticity, so will your lungs, liver, heart, stomach and kidneys gain in efficiency and productivity.

When you exercise regularly, the arch of your ribs widens. This gives free play to your lungs. Your elastic diaphragm allows the heart to pump and function more powerfully. Your rubberlike waist, in its limber action, stimulates your kidneys and massages your liver. Your abdominal muscles strengthen and support your stomach with controlled undulations. All this trunk exercise acts like a massage of the vital organs and exerts an influence over the whole organism that must not be underestimated – it's so vital for your Super Health!

Should We Exercise During Fasting?

Only the faster can answer this question. If there is no inclination for physical activity during a fast, then don't exercise. At most do some relaxing stretches and deep breathing. The fast is giving you a physiological rest. Unless you have a big urge for physical activity, you should relax and rest as much as possible when fasting.

During a fast, your body is using all of its Vital Force for internal purification, but if during a 7 to 10 day fast you feel the need for some stretching or walking, respond to the urge. It is between fasts and in your daily program of living that you should spend a portion of every day of your life exercising, preferably outdoors. Soon you will enjoy a vigorous circulation instead of a sluggish one. Poor circulation causes many health problems, discomfort, pain and misery throughout the body.

Don't injure your body by over-eating. It will kill you before your time.

Fasting is cleansing, purifying and restful. – Meir Schneider

Fasting & Exercise Promotes Health & Energy

The more you fast, the more poisons you cleanse from your body. As your body increases its internal cleanliness, your muscles will enjoy more energy, tone and vitality. You will find that your old, sluggish, lazy feelings will leave you and you will desire more action and more physical activity. Life will become more exciting!

When people don't exercise, their ankles and legs often swell because there's not enough blood circulating to remove the waste from the cells and carry it back to the organs of elimination. Allow no excuses for not exercising! Regardless of your physical condition, it's vitally important that some form of exercise become a part of your Bragg Healthy Lifestyle. Plan and get started.

Exercise helps avert sickness and premature ageing! It builds a health fund of endurance and resistance. It helps to build a healthy bloodstream with properly balanced white and red corpuscles that help keep us healthy by keeping our immune system on constant guard to fight off any germs, illnesses, etc.

Exercise helps maintain a serene and tranquil mind and increases confidence. A one to three mile walk in the fresh air with God and Mother Nature helps neutralize most all unhealthful emotional upsets. The knowledge that you have improved your mental and physical abilities through exercise will give you supreme confidence. Exercise helps cultivate will power and gives you control of your Physical, Mental and Spiritual Self which helps you to further promote your personal efficiency, happiness and longevity.

Exercise is the greatest health tonic we can provide ourselves! To attain this feeling of radiant, glorious health, follow The Bragg Healthy Lifestyle and engage in regular, vigorous physical activity. You will look and feel better and more youthful! This lifestyle will produce miraculous feelings of radiant, joyous agelessness.

Studies show it is never too late to begin exercising. Recent physical activity has a greater positive impact on health and cardiovascular disease and mortality than exercise done in one's past. – Sports Medicine Digest

Do these Exercises Daily (10 per set):

You must exercise! It's important because weak muscles of the arms, legs and entire body indicates a similar unhealthy condition also of the stomach muscles and heart (a muscle) and other organs.

Important Exercises for Keeping the External and Internal Muscles of The Stomach Fit and Healthy. These Also Promote Good Elimination and Energy.

Bend at the waist to the sides, then front and back.

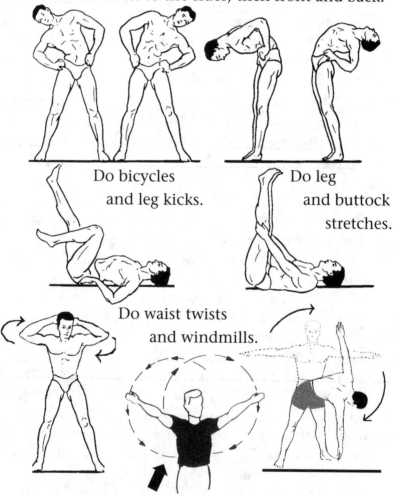

Do bicycles and leg kicks.

Do leg and buttock stretches.

Do waist twists and windmills.

Windmill Exercise: *Swing arms forward and go around in large circles. Let your hands feel heavy and let the hands carry your arms around and around. Now do backward circles. Breathe easily and deeply, feet 10 inches apart, bend your knees a little and then straighten them up with each circle. Do 5 to 10 times daily. Results: tension goes, energy increases!*

THE MIRACLES OF APPLE CIDER VINEGAR FOR A STRONGER, LONGER, HEALTHIER LIFE

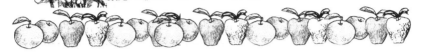

The old adage is true:
"An apple a day keeps the doctor away."

- Helps promote a youthful skin and vibrant healthy body
- Helps remove artery plaque and body toxins
- Helps fight germs, viruses, bacteria and mold naturally
- Helps retard old age onset in humans, pets and farm animals
- Helps regulate calcium metabolism
- Helps keep blood the right consistency
- Helps regulate women's menstruation and relieves PMS
- Helps normalize urine pH, relieving frequent urge to urinate
- Helps digestion, assimilation and balances the pH
- Helps relieve sore throats, laryngitis and throat tickles and cleans out throat and gum toxins
- Helps detox the body so sinus, asthma and flu sufferers can breathe easier and more normally
- Helps banish acne, athlete's foot, soothes burns, sunburns
- Helps relieve itching scalp, baldness, dry hair and banishes dandruff, rashes, and shingles
- Helps fight arthritis and removes crystals and toxins from joints, tissues, organs and entire body
- Helps control and normalize body weight

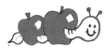

– Paul C. Bragg, Health Crusader,
Originator of Health Food Stores
– 3 John 2 –

Our sincere blessings to you, **dear friends,** who make our lives so worthwhile and fulfilled by reading our teachings on natural living as our Creator laid down for us to follow. He wants us to follow the simple path of natural living. This is what we teach in our books and health crusades worldwide. Our prayers reach out to you and your loved ones for the best in health and happiness. We must follow the laws He has laid down for us, so we can reap this precious health physically, mentally, emotionally and spiritually!

HAVE AN APPLE HEALTHY LIFE!

With Love, ~Patricia Bragg~

Braggs Organic Raw Apple Cider Vinegar with the "Mother Enzyme" is the #1 food I recommend to maintain the body's vital acid – alkaline balance.
– Gabriel Cousens, M.D., Author, *Conscious Eating*

Vitamin D is Important for Bones, Teeth & Health!

Vitamin D is a hormone and like other hormones it is manufactured in the body. It helps the body utilize calcium and phosphorus and builds bones and teeth. Recent studies show that _vitamin D inhibits the growth of cancer cells, including those in the breast and prostate_. Statistics from a California survey of American women found women with higher sun exposure and those with a high dietary intake of vitamin D, sun-grown foods, etc. had lower risk of breast cancer. A University of North Carolina study also found the same results. Evidence also points to a link between vitamin D and reduced risk of colon cancer.

Small amounts of gentle sunlight on your skin cells causes them to manufacture vitamin D. Even as little as 10 to 15 minutes, 2 to 3 times a week should be sufficient to meet your needs. Sunscreen can reduce or even shut down the synthesis of vitamin D, so we recommend exposure to gentle early morning or late afternoon rays without the use of sunscreen. If needed, apply sunscreen (SPF 30 for UVA/UVB.) when in sun longer, especially if fair-skinned. Those under 50 need 200 IUs, 50-70 need 400 IUs and those over 70 need 600 IUs of vitamin D daily and more in special cases. Older people's ability declines to produce vitamin D from sunlight. That's why it's important for those over 70 to get vitamin D from supplements and foods: wheat germ, raw sunflower seeds, cod liver oil, sweet potatoes, corn bread, eggs, alfalfa, saltwater fish, sardines, salmon, tuna, liver and natural vegetable oils are good sources of vitamin D.

Vitamin D is a major protective factor guarding against chemical sensitivities and infections. Cod liver oil which parents once gave automatically to children is a an excellent preventive medicine, with its high concentrations of vitamins A and D. – Dr. Michael Schachter, Columbia University
www.mbschachter.com

Sunflower seeds are sun-energized and have vitamin D partially due to the flower's tendency to follow and face the sun as it moves across the sky. Raw sunflower seeds are one of the few vegetable sources for vitamin D. They are delicious for salads, pep-drinks, cookies, breads, trail mix snacks, etc. and try sunflower sprouts for salads.

IMPORTANT HEALTH FACTS!

Scientists at the Department of Agriculture's Human Nutrition Research Center on Ageing in Boston report that daily requirements for vitamins B-6, B-12, C, D and E escalate with age, along with the need for calcium, beta carotene and folic acid. Play it safe – be sure to take natural multi-vitamin and mineral supplements.

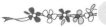 **AN OLD ENGLISH PRAYER**

Give us Lord, a bit of sun, a bit of work and a bit of fun.
Give us, in all struggle and sputter, our daily whole grain bread and food.
Give us health, our keep to make and a bit to spare for others' sake.
Give us too, a bit of song and a tale and a book, to help us along.
Give us Lord, a chance to be our goodly best for ourselves and others,
Until men learn to live as brothers in peace and harmony.

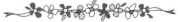

Giving and receiving love makes everyday a honeymoon! – Patricia Bragg

Chapter 23

Doctor Gentle Sunshine

Doctor Sunshine's specialty is heliotherapy and his great prescription is solar energy. Each tiny blade of grass, every vine, tree, bush, flower, fruit and vegetable draws its life from solar energy. All living things on earth depend on solar energy for their existence. The earth would be a barren, frigid place if it were not for the magic rays of the sun! The sun gives us light, and were it not for light, there would be no you or me. Earth would be in total darkness and void of life. (We endorse solar energy when possible).

A person's skin is gently tanned by the sun and air and will take on a darker pigment according to its original type. It has been found that with gentle exposure to the sun even redheaded people will eventually tan. Pigmentation is a sign that solar energy has been transformed into human energy. Mankind can gain health, vitality and happiness in the gentle, healing rays of the sun.

The people who are indoors too long have sallow, ghostly-looking skin. That is why so many women hide their sun-starved skins with face makeup. People who are deprived of the vital rays of the sun have a half-dead look. They are actually dying for want of solar energy! Weak, ailing, anemic people are usually sun-starved and, in our opinion, many people are sick simply because they are starving for sunshine.

The rays of the sun are powerful germicides. As the skin imbibes more of these rays, it stores up enormous amounts of this germ-killing energy. The gentle sun provides a remedy for the nervous person filled with anxiety, worry, stresses and strains. When these tense people lie in the early morning or late afternoon gentle sunshine, its healing rays give them what the nerves and body are crying out for . . . and that is relaxation!

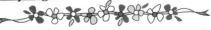

What sculpture is to a block of marble, education is to the mind and soul.
– Addison, The Spectator

Chlorophyll is Miracle Liquid Sunshine

Gentle sunshine is a soothing tonic, a stimulant and above all, the Great Healer! As you bask in the warm, gentle sunshine (not the hot afternoon sun), millions of nerve endings absorb the energy from the sun and transform it so the body's nervous system can use it.

Perform this experiment to determine the value of sunshine in the matter of life and death. Find a beautiful lawn, where the grass is like a green carpet. Cover up a small space of that beautiful lawn with a piece of wood or a small box. Day by day you will notice that the beautiful grass that once was full of plant blood, precious chlorophyll, will fade and turn a sickly yellow. Tragically, it withers and dies – death by sun starvation! The same thing happens in your body without the sun's life-giving rays and without an abundance of sun-ripened foods such as organic fruits, vegetables and their fresh juices.

We must have the direct gentle rays of the sun on our bodies and at least 60% to 70% percent of the food we eat must have been ripened by the sun's rays. When we eat fresh, organically grown fruits and vegetables, we absorb the blood of the plant – chlorophyll. This life-giving chlorophyll is the solar energy that the plant has absorbed from the sun, the richest, most nourishing food you can put in your body. Green plants and vegetables alone possess the secret of how to capture this powerful solar energy and pass it on to man and every other living creature. When you put sunshine on the outside of your body and eat ample sun-grown, organic fruits and vegetables, you are going to glow with more super health! But these powerful, natural remedies must be taken in small doses at the beginning, because your sun-starved body can't absorb too much at first.

Gentle Sunbathing Works Miracles!

When you begin sunbathing, start with short time periods until you condition your body to take more. The best time for beginners to start taking 10 and 15 minute sunbaths is in the early morning sunshine until 10 a.m. or late afternoon sunshine after 3 p.m. Between 11 and 3 we usually avoid stronger, burning rays. (*We wear straw hats.*)

154

The same caution should be taken when eating the sun-ripened raw fruits and vegetables. The average person who has been eating mainly cooked foods will find that if great amounts of raw fruits and vegetables suddenly enter into the body they can cause a reaction. It's wiser to gradually add more sun-ripened foods to the diet. Overdoses of solar energy, both outside and inside the body, are not wise. Regarding sun exposure, use good judgment and caution. For sun (skin) protection when needed make a green (non-caffeine) tea and apply to skin.)

Doctor Healing Sunshine Saved Bragg's Life!

When my father was diagnosed with tuberculosis at 16, three TB Sanitariums later the best TB doctors in the USA declared his case *hopeless and incurable!* Yet, by the grace of God, he was led to Dr. August Rollier of Leysin, Switzerland, the greatest living authority on heliotherapy (sun cure). High in the Swiss Alps, Dad's sick and wasted body was exposed to the gentle healing rays of the sun and fed an abundance of natural, sun-ripened foods.

A healing miracle happened. In just two years he was transformed from a hopeless invalid on his deathbed to a vitally strong young man who radiated health! At 95 years young he was still healthy, happy and powerful. Throughout these years, he enjoyed the great outdoors and the healing rays of the gentle sun on his body.

That is why my father and I have always loved God's own precious sunshine. That's why we made our main home in California, the great sunshine state. We have an organic farm in Santa Barbara near the ocean where we get the benefits of the clean air and sunshine. We also live part-time in Hawaii so we can visit with the Bragg readers who visit our free Bragg Exercise Class (pg. i) at famous Waikiki Beach. The class is 6 days a week and such fun to exercise in the fresh clean air. We enjoy our students who come from all over the world. Seek fresh, clean air, gentle sunshine and organic sun-kissed foods, then soon super health will leap out and be yours to treasure throughout a long, ever youthful, productive, life!

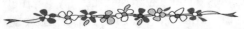

God gave His creatures light and air and water open to the skies; Man locks himself in a stifling lair and wonders why his brother dies. – Oliver W. Holmes

Locations in the Body Where Osteoporosis, Arthritis, Pain and Misery Hit the Hardest

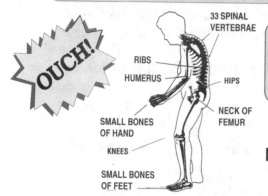

OUCH!

33 SPINAL VERTEBRAE
RIBS
HUMERUS
HIPS
NECK OF FEMUR
SMALL BONES OF HAND
KNEES
SMALL BONES OF FEET

OSTEOPOROSIS
Affects over 30 Million and Kills 400,000 Americans Annually

Boron
Miracle Trace Mineral For Healthy Bones

BORON – A trace mineral for healthier bones that also helps the body absorb more vital calcium, minerals and necessary hormones! Good sources are most vegetables, fresh and sun- dried fruits, prunes, raw nuts, soybeans and nutritional Brewer's yeast. The U.S. Department of Agriculture's Human Nutrition Lab in Grand Forks, North Dakota, says boron is usually found in soil and in foods, but many Americans eat a diet low in boron. They conducted a 17 week study which showed a daily 3 to 6 mgs boron supplement enabled participants to reduce loss (demineralization) of calcium, phosphorus and magnesium from their bodies. This loss is usually caused by eating refined, processed, fast foods and lots of meat, salt, sugar and fat and a dietary lack of fresh vegetables, fruits and whole grains. *(Visit-www.all-natural.com)*

After 8 weeks on boron, participants' calcium loss was cut 40%. It also helped double important hormone levels vital in maintaining calcium and healthy bones. (Rutgers Study says 1,700mg of calcium from food & supplements is important after menopause). Millions of women on estrogen therapy for osteoporosis* may want to use boron, a healthier choice. Also consider natural progesterone (2%) raw yam cream and other natural options. For pain, joint support and healing, use a glucosamine/chondriotin/MSM combo *(caps, liquid and roll-on)*.

University of Wales recent study showed Cod Liver Oil eases pain and heals. Scientific studies also show women benefit from a healthy lifestyle that includes some gentle sunshine and ample exercise *(even weightlifting)* to maintain healthier bones, combined with a low-fat, high-fiber, natural carbohydrates and fresh salads, greens, vegetable, fruit diet and also add ½ tsp cinnamon powder to teas, drinks, etc. This lifestyle helps protect against heart disease, high blood pressure, cancer and many other ailments. I'm happy to see science now agrees with my Dad who first stated these health truths over 80 years ago!

156

* *For more hormone and osteoporosis facts read pioneer Dr. John Lee's book. What Your Doctor May Not Tell You About Menopause. www.amazon.com*

Chapter 24

Alternative Health Therapies And Massage Techniques

Try Them – They Work Miracles!

Explore these wonderful natural methods of healing your body. Then choose the best healing techniques for you:

ACUPUNCTURE/ACUPRESSURE Acupuncture directs and rechannels body energy by inserting hair-thin needles (use only disposable needles) at specific points on the body. It's used for pain, backaches, migraines and general health and body dysfunctions. Used in Asia for centuries, acupuncture is safe, virtually painless and has no side effects. **Acupressure** is based on the same principles and uses finger pressure and massage rather than needles. Websites offer info, check them out. Web: *acupuncture.com*

CHIROPRACTIC Chiropractic was founded in Davenport, Iowa in 1885 by Daniel David Palmer. There are now many schools in the U.S., and graduates are joining Health Practitioners in all nations of the world to share healing techniques. Chiropractic is popular, is the largest U.S. healing profession benefitting literally millions. Treatment involves soft tissue, spinal and body adjustment to free the nervous system of interferences with normal body function. Its concern is the functional integrity of the musculoskeletal system. In addition to manual methods, chiropractors use physical therapy modalities, exercise, health and nutritional guidance. Web: *chiropractic.org*

F. MATHIUS ALEXANDER TECHNIQUE These lessons help end improper use of neuromuscular system and bring body posture back into balance. Eliminates psycho-physical interferences, helps release long-held tension, and aids in re-establishing muscle tone. Web: alexandertechnique.com

FELDENKRAIS METHOD Dr. Moshe Feldenkrais founded this in the 1940s. Lessons lead to improved posture and help create ease and efficiency of body movement. This is a great stress removal method. Web: *feldenkrais.com*

The physician must be experienced in many things, but most assuredly in healing, soothing massages. – Hippocrates, Father of Medicine 400 B.C.

Alternative Health Therapies & Massage Techniques

HOMEOPATHY In the 1800's, Dr. Samuel Hahnemann developed homeopathy. Patients are treated with minute amounts of substances similar to those that cause a particular disease to trigger the body's own defenses. The homeopathic principle is *Like Cures Like*. This safe and nontoxic remedy is the #1 alternative therapy in Europe and Britain because it is inexpensive, seldom has any side effects, and brings fast results. Web: *www.homeopathy.org*

NATUROPATHY Brought to America by pioneer Dr. Benedict Lust, M.D., this treatment uses diet, herbs, homeopathy, fasting, exercise, hydrotherapy, manipulation and sunlight. (Dr. Paul C. Bragg graduated from Dr. Lust's first School of Naturopathy in U.S., Now there's 6 schools.) Practitioners work with your body to restore health naturally. They reject surgery and drugs except as a last resort. Web:*www.pandamedicine.com*

OSTEOPATHY The first School of Osteopathy was founded in 1892 by Dr. Andrew Taylor Still, M.D. There are now 15 U.S. colleges. Treatment involves soft tissue, spinal and body adjustments that free the nervous system from interferences that can cause illness. Healing by adjustment also includes physical therapies, good nutrition, proper breathing and good posture. Dr. Still's premise: if the body structure is altered or abnormal, then proper body function is altered and can cause pain and illness. Web: *osteopathy.org*

REFLEXOLOGY OR ZONE THERAPY Founded by Eunice Ingham, author of *Stories The Feet Can Tell*, inspired by a Bragg Health Crusade when she was 17. Reflexology helps the body by removing crystalline deposits from reflex areas (nerve endings) of feet and hands through deep pressure massage. Reflexology originated in China and Egypt and Native American Indians and Kenyans practiced it for centuries. Reflexology activates the body's flow of healing and energy by dislodging deposits. Visit Eunice Ingham's website at *www.reflexology-usa.net* and *www.reflexology.org*

SKIN BRUSHING daily is wonderful for circulation, toning, cleansing and healing. Use a dry vegetable brush (never nylon) and brush lightly. Helps purify lymph so it's able to detoxify your blood and tissues. Removes old skin cells, uric acid crystals and toxic wastes that come up through skin's pores. Use loofah sponge for variety in shower or tub.

Alternative Health Therapies & Massage Techniques

REIKI A Japanese form of massage that means "Universal Life Energy." Reiki helps the body to detoxify, then re-balance and heal itself. Discovered in the ancient Sutra manuscripts by Dr. Mikso Usui in 1822. Web: *reiki.com*

ROLFING Developed by Ida Rolf in the 1930's in the U.S. Rolfing is also called structural processing and postural release, or structural dynamics. It is based on the concept that distortions (accidents, injuries, falls, etc.) and the effects of gravity on the body cause upsets in the body. Rolfing helps to achieve balance and improved body posture. Methods involve the use of stretching, deep tissue massage, and relaxation techniques to loosen old injuries and break bad movement and posture patterns, which can cause long-term health and body stress. Web: *rolf.org*

TRAGERING Founded by Dr. Milton Trager M.D., who was inspired at age 18 by Paul C. Bragg to become a doctor. It is an experimental learning method that involves gentle shaking and rocking, suggesting a greater letting go, releasing tensions and lengthening of muscles for more body health. Tragering can do miraculous healing where needed in the muscles and the entire body. Web: *trager.com*

WATER THERAPY Soothing detox shower: apply olive oil to skin, alternate hot and cold water. Massage areas while under hot, filtered spray (pages 130-132). Garden hose massage is great in summer. Hot detox tub bath (20 minutes) with cup each of Epsom salts and apple cider vinegar, pulls out toxins by creating an artificial fever cleanse. Web: *nmsnt.org*

MASSAGE & AROMATHERAPY works two ways: the essence (aroma) relaxes, as does the massage. Essential oils are extracted from flowers, leaves, roots, seeds and barks. These are usually massaged into the skin, inhaled or used in a bath for their ability to relax, soothe and heal. The oils, used for centuries to treat numerous ailments, are revitalizing and energizing for the body and mind. Example: Tiger balm, MSM, echinacea and arnica help relieve muscle aches. Avoid skin creams and lotions with mineral oil – it clogs the skin's pores. Use these natural oils for the skin: almond, apricot kernel, avocado, soy, hemp seed and olive oils and mix with aromatic essential oils: rosemary, lavender, rose, jasmine, sandalwood, lemon-balm, etc. –6 oz. oil & 6 drops of an essential oil. Web: *aromatherapy.com* or *frontierherb.com*

159

Alternative Health Therapies & Massage Techniques

MASSAGE – SELF Paul C. Bragg often said, "You can be your own best massage therapist, even if you have only one good hand." Near-miraculous health improvements have been achieved by victims of accidents or strokes in bringing life back to afflicted parts of their own bodies by self-massage and even vibrators. Treatments can be day or night, almost continual. Self-massage also helps achieve relaxation at day's end. Families and friends can learn and exchange massages; it's a wonderful sharing experience. Remember, babies also love and thrive with daily massages, start from birth. Family pets also love the soothing, healing touch of massages. Web: *amtamassage.org*

MASSAGE – SHIATSU Japanese form of health massage that applies pressure from the fingers, hands, elbows and even knees along the same points as acupuncture. Shiatsu has been used in Asia for centuries to relieve pain, common ills, body and muscle stress and aids lymphatic circulation.

MASSAGE – SPORTS An important health support system for professional and amateur athletes. Sports massage improves circulation and mobility to injured tissue, enables athletes to recover more rapidly from myofascial injury, reduces muscle soreness and chronic strain patterns. Soft tissues are freed of trigger points and adhesions, thus contributing to improvement of peak neuro-muscular functioning and athletic performance.

MASSAGE – SWEDISH One of the oldest and most popular and widely used massage techniques. This deep body massage soothes and promotes circulation and is also a great way to loosen and relax muscles before and after exercise.

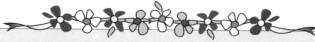

Author's Comment: We have personally sampled many of these alternative therapies. It's estimated that soon America's health care costs will leap over $2 trillion. It's more important than ever to be responsible for our own health! This includes seeking holistic health practitioners who are dedicated to keeping us well by inspiring us to practice prevention! These Alternative Healing Therapies are also popular and getting results: aroma, Ayurvedic, biofeedback, color, guided imagery, herbs, music, meditation, magnets, saunas, tai chi, chi gong, Pilates, yoga, etc. Explore them and be open to improving your earthly temple for a healthier, happier, longer life. **Seek and find the best for your body, mind and soul.** – **Patricia Bragg**

What wound did ever heal but by gentle degrees. – William Shakespeare

Chapter 25

Health Alternatives to
Help With Breathing Problems

- Massage • Acupuncture • Chiropractic
- Herbs • Exercise • Nutrition • Water

Don't Accept Breathing Problems – Solve Them

The healthiest, best thing to do instead of taking drugs for asthma, sinus, bronchitis and breathing problems is to seek natural remedies to correct any problems. <u>Drugs should never be the main method of seeking a cure</u>. These drugs and applications are commonly called "maintenance drugs". Even this is misleading because the problems they supposedly relieve often get worse over time. Not to mention the many other side effects they have on the entire body!

The three prominent types of drugs for sinus problems in the medical field are: bronchodilators, anti-inflammatories and antihistamines. Although the first two of these can supply some relief during attacks by opening narrowed breathing pathways, they are very dangerous and ill-advised. A study of bronchodilators (drug puffers) in New Zealand found that their habit forming use brought an increased risk of asthma-related deaths and injury. Antihistamines, on the other hand, really promise no relief to asthma sufferers, even in the short-term. Their effect is merely to dry up mucus secretions and replace the aggravating plugs of thick mucus with dried, clogging crusts of mucus.

For a healthy nose, it's essential to live The Bragg Healthy Lifestyle. Practice this lifestyle formula for good physical and mental health. A healthy head and body are necessary preconditions to a healthy, happy nose!

According to recent medical studies more people suffer from a condition called multiple chemical sensitivity. Now it is more crucial that you and your family practice natural healthy living habits to stay healthy!

Pollution and Wrong Diet Affects Breathing

In addition, if you live in a polluted area, or if your sinuses are already damaged from the hard work of protecting your lungs, buy a high-efficiency, charcoal particulate HEPA air filtration system. This pre-filters the air your sinuses will filter, making your nose's job easier. Also have one for your home, office and car.

You must also be intelligent about your allergies. If you know you are allergic to particular substances, take precautions to avoid them. If you suspect allergies, take the necessary steps to learn what's affecting you. The most common allergens are mold spores, animal hair and dander, toxic house dust, mites, pollens and even carpet and paint chemicals, etc. Food allergies are also a frequent source of allergic respiratory reactions. (See page 32.)

With long-term relief in mind, stay informed about the effective alternative therapies available today. The most sensible therapy to practice, no matter what the health complaint, is **Nutritional Therapy**. When it comes to sinus problems it's most important to avoid dairy products of all kinds. Dairy foods are unhealthy for the nose and the whole body. Dairy proteins often mimic allergens by causing the nose and throat airway passages to swell. They also increase mucus production. This in turn causes sinus discomfort and can give rise to dangerous bacterial conditions. If you are a snorer or a sufferer of any sinus condition you will especially benefit from a no-dairy diet. Try it – prove it to yourself!

In addition to healthy living and avoiding all dairy, you can relieve sinusitis symptoms and bolster the health of your nose by using **Herbal Therapy** such as: licorice, anise and horehound, brigham tea, mint, echinacea, fenugreek, goldenseal, lobelia, marshmallow, mullein, red clover and rose hips. Herbs are available in teas, capsules or tablets. Medicinal herbs, soaked in a cloth poultice (warm), can provide relief for sore, congested areas. (Example: old fashion mustard pack for chest colds.)

If you truly love Nature, you will find Beauty everywhere. – Van Gogh

Healing Therapy & Healthy Lifestyle, Works Miracles

Chiropractic Therapy has shown to provide relief by stimulating the nerves that control the lungs. The nerves that send messages to the lungs are located on the spine just below the neck and can be manipulated for increased stimulation. These procedures can also have beneficial effects on the diaphragm. Some practitioners can even make adjustments on some of the small bones and cartilage of the nose for increased breathing comfort.

For many thousands of years *Acupuncture Therapy* has been used in Asia. It often helps to relieve the complaints of asthma and sinus. The professional placement of needles (disposable) often can provide relief from airway spasms and encourage passages to dilate, permitting greater flow of air.

Many techniques of ***Massage and Pressure-Pointing Therapy*** can bring relief for the asthmatic. Among the various disciplines, **Shiatsu Therapy** has become popular for the victims of sinus discomfort. Although it bears some similarity to needle acupuncture, Shaitsu uses finger-pressure, like *Acupressure Therapy* to stimulate the body's own rehabilitative functions.

No matter what therapies you practice, consider **Water Therapy** as essential! Never fail to drink at least 8 tall glasses of pure distilled water every day. This will help your mucus membranes and sinuses efficiently filter and dispose of the contaminants that pollute our air. Throughout this book we have continued to inform you of all the various health alternatives for your health!

Caring hands have healing lifeforce energy . . . babies love and thrive with daily massages and cuddles. Family pets love soothing, healing touches. Everyone benefits from healing massages and treatments! – Patricia Bragg

---

There is no trifling with nature; it is always true, dignified, and just; it is always in the right, and the faults and errors belong to us. Nature defies incompetence, but reveals its secrets to the competent, the truthful, and the pure. – Johann W. Goethe

---

Living under conditions of modern life, it's important to bear in mind that the refinement, overprocessing & cooking of food products either entirely eliminates or partly destroys the vital elements in the original material.
– United States Department of Agriculture – www.usda.gov

Health is Your Birthright – Protect and Treasure It!

This is a priceless book. Please read and re-read this book until you absorb every health nugget it contains. Remember that you and you alone control your life, your health and the way you look, act, think and feel! Health comes from the inside out. You can be patched up after being stricken with disease, sickness and physical pain, but 100% true, robust, vital health comes from good *health habits!* This book shows you how to turn away from the damaging, unhealthy lifestyle habits that careless, wrong living promotes.

It is up to you to apply the intelligence that our Creator gave you. We teach simple, healthy living. You now have a treasure of knowledge of how to create a healthier, more joyful life through living this simple, healthy lifestyle. Have faith in yourself, start now!

Your health depends on your total lifestyle . . . the way you conduct yourself each hour, each day, each week, each month and each year. You are the sum total of your habits! It is true that your body can take a lot of punishment from your bad habits. Sure, you can smoke, drink, eat dead, devitalized foods and apparently look and feel fine. Yes, for a while . . . but sooner or later you will have to balance your debts with Mother Nature! And when something breaks and you have heart trouble or one of hundreds of other life and health destroying miseries, it may be too late! It may mean years of living death – or it may mean quick death.

We have no supernatural power to prevent or cure disease. That power is in your body. Your body is self-cleansing and self-healing when given a chance. We can only come to you as health teachers, to tell you in a simple way what living this healthy lifestyle will do for you. You have the knowledge; it's now up to you to apply the intelligence that our Creator gave you! **Living The Bragg Healthy Lifestyle is simply good common sense.**

Knowing these teachings will mean true life and good health for you.
– Proverbs 4:22

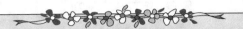

Earn Your Bragging Rights

Live The Bragg Healthy Lifestyle To Attain Supreme Physical, Mental, Emotional and Spiritual Health!

With your new awareness, understanding and sincere commitment of how to live The Bragg Healthy Lifestyle – you can now live a longer, healthier life to 120 years!

God bless you and your family and may He give you the strength, the courage and the patience to win your battle to re-enter the Healthy Garden of Eden while you are still living here on Earth with time to enjoy it all!

With Blessings of Health, Peace, Joy and Love,

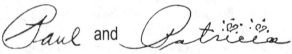

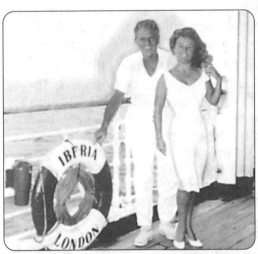

Health Crusaders Paul C. Bragg and daughter Patricia traveled the world spreading health, inspiring millions to renew and revitalize their health.
- 3 John 2
- Genesis 6:3

The Bragg books are written to inspire and guide you to health, fitness and longevity. Remember, the book you don't read won't help. So please read and reread the Bragg Books and live The Bragg Healthy Lifestyle!

I never suspected that I would have to learn how to live – that there were specific disciplines and ways of seeing the world that I had to master before I could awaken to a simple, healthy, happy, uncomplicated life.
– Dan Millman, Author of The Way of the Peaceful Warrior - www.danmillman.com
A Bragg fan and admirer since Stanford University coaching days.

A truly good book teaches me better than to just read it,
I must soon lay it down and commence living in its wisdom.
What I began by reading, I must finish by acting! – Henry David Thoreau

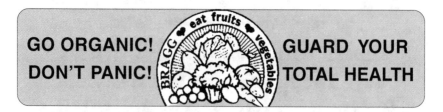

**GO ORGANIC!
DON'T PANIC!** eat fruits • vegetables BRAGG **GUARD YOUR
TOTAL HEALTH**

FROM THE AUTHORS

This book was written for You! It can be your passport to a healthy, long, vital life. We in the Alternative Health Therapies join hands in one common objective – promoting a high standard of health for everyone. Healthy nutrition points the way – which is Mother Nature and God's Way. This book teaches you how to work with them, not against them. Health Doctors, therapists nurses, teachers and caregivers are becoming more dedicated than ever before to keeping their patients healthy and fit. This book was written to emphasize the greatly needed importance of living a lifetime of healthy living, close to Mother Nature and God.

Statements in this book are scientific health findings, known facts of physiology and biological therapeutics. Paul C. Bragg practiced natural methods of living for over 80 years with highly beneficial results, knowing that they were safe and of great value. His daughter Patricia lectured and co-authored the Bragg Books with him and continues to carrying on The Bragg Health Crusades.

Paul C. Bragg and daughter Patricia express their opinions solely as Public Health Educators and Health Crusaders. They offer no cure for disease. Only the body has the ability to cure a person. Experts may disagree with some of the statements made in this book. However, such statements are considered to be factual, based on the long-time health experience of pioneers Paul C. Bragg and Patricia Bragg. If you suspect you have a medical problem, please seek alternative health professionals to help you make the healthiest, wisest and best-informed choices.

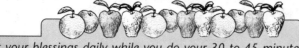

Count your blessings daily while you do your 30 to 45 minute brisk walks and exercises with these affirmations – health! strength! youth! vitality! peace! laughter! humility! understanding! forgiveness! joy! and love for eternity! – and soon all these qualities will come flooding and bouncing into your life. With blessings of super health, peace and love to you, our dear friends – our readers. – Patricia Bragg

If I were to name the three most precious resources of life, I would say books, friends and nature; and the greatest of these, at least the most constant and always at hand is nature and God. – John Burroughs

Peace is not a season, it is a way of life.

Change your mind and you change your life.

Index

A

Abdomen, 27, 42, 50, 59, 148
Acupressure, 163
Acupuncture, 163
Adrenaline, 108
Aerobic exercise, 77, 86, 137
Ageing, 4-6, 98, 121, 126,
   137-138, 149, 152
Air, clean 17-18, 30, 35-39, 65
   91-95
Air baths, 65-66, 136
Air filters/fans, 18, 63, 95
Air passages, 78, 81, 95, 129
Air pollution, 30, 35, 79, 91-95
Air lung sacs, 11, 16-17, 19-20,
   41, 57, 70, 81
Alexander Technique, 157
Allergies, 32-33, 40, 95, 120, 162
Anger, 13
Animal dander, 17, 82, 162
Anticoagulant, 145
Aorta, 8, 11, 71
Apple Cider Vinegar, 64, 78, 82,
   101, 105-106, 114-116, 141, 151
Aromatherapy, 80, 143, 159
Aromatic Massage, 159
Arteries 10-11, 43, 50
Arteriosclerosis, 108
Arthritis, 111-112, 119, 156
Asthma, 6, 79, 81-82, 129, 161
Athletes, 54, 62, 97, 136
ATP (adenosine triphosphate), 84
Auto-intoxication, 12
Ayurveda Therapy, 40, 44-45

B

Babies, 4, 23, 41, 84
Backaches, 6, 47-50, 78
Basal Metabolism, 9
Bedtime Routines, 73, 80
Beverages, 107, 116
Birth, 84, 133
Blood, 7-13, 16, 18-20, 23, 27 43,
   56, 63-64, 71, 74-76, 84, 101,
   111, 115, 121, 124-125, 133, 135,
   138-139, 145, 149, 167
Bones, 112, 124, 156
Boron, 156
Bowels, 26, 59, 69
Bragg Health Crusade, 20, 159
Bragg Posture Exercise, 52, 58, 85
Bragg Super Power Breathing
   exercises, 59-71, 74-75, 83-90
Brain, 4, 7, 13-14, 17, 64, 68-69
Bras, 52
Breads, 99, 119, 121
Breathing, 4, 15
Broken bones, 124
Bronchitis, 6, 79, 81-82, 161
Buildings, unhealthy, 35-38
Burns, 98

C

Caffeine (coffee), 19, 80
Calcium, 80, 110, 112-113, 152
Calisthenics, 77, 147
Cancer, 19, 96, 100, 101
Capillaries, 10-11, 16, 47
Carbon Dioxide, 7, 10, 14, 74

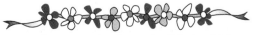

When you sell a man a book you don't just sell him paper,
ink and glue, you sell him a whole new life! – Christopher Morley

Remember: "It is NEVER too late to be what you might have been!"

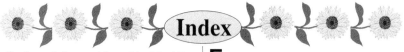

Carbon Monoxide, 19, 22, 37

Cardiovascular, 19-29, 34, 37, 98

Cartilage, 16, 29, 163

Cells, 9, 11, 64, 133

Childbirth, 84

Chiropractic, 157, 161, 163

Chlorophyll, 154

Cholesterol, 10, 108, 138, 145
   Healthy Heart Habits, 138

Circulatory System, 8-9, 161

Cleansing, 12, 25-27, 74, 114, 120

Cleansing Breath, 67

Clothing, loose, 52-53, 139-140

Cold-water swimming, 53

Common cold, 25-27

Complexion, 13, 55

Concentration, 13-14

Constipation, 6, 12, 43, 146

Contaminants, 18, 24, 30, 60

Cornmeal Recipe, 99

D

Dancers, 54 - 55

Decongestants, 31, 81

Diaphragm, 15, 41-44, 47, 55-60,
   67, 69, 74, 82-83, 148

Diaphragmatic Breathing, 42-44

Diarrhea, 26

Diet, 12, 101, 105-123

Digestive Tract, 125

Dinner, 107

Distilled water, 26, 74, 101, 106,
   112, 115-116, 120-121, 142

Doctor Exercise, 145-150

Doctor Fresh Air, 133-138

Doctor Good Posture, 47-56

Doctor Rest, 139-144

Doctor Sunshine, 153-155

E

Elimination, 6, 12, 43, 69, 146

Emotions, 1, 13, 50, 78

Emphysema, 6, 19, 79

Energy, 1-4, 9-10, 44, 50, 54-58,
   62-65, 72-73, 77, 95, 101, 105,
   107, 114, 134, 137, 139, 142,
   144, 147, 149, 153-155, 157,
   159, 163, 174

Exercise, 2-3, 7, 10-11, 25, 27,
   34, 40, 42-45, 48, 50, 52,
   55-60, 62-77, 82-83, 97, 105
   105, 116, 125, 133, 136, 138, 141-
   150, 157, 161, 166, 176-177

Extrasensory perception, 14

Eyes, 6, 12, 24, 29, 36, 56

F

Fasting, 105, 114, 117, 120
   136, 148, 159

Fatigue, 44, 52, 76

Feet, 74-75, 139

Feldenkrais Method, 131

Fever, 26

Fiber chart, 122

Filters, 18, 32, 60, 95

Flu, 24, 26, 78, 163

Fluoride, 112, 115

Food Allergies, 32-34, 40, 95, 120,

Foods to Avoid list, 121

Fruits, 68, 101-103

G

Gallbladder, 43, 115

Gardening, 117, 147

Gout, 54, 74

Gums, 6, 126

Until you make peace with who you are, you'll never
be content with what you have – Doris Mortman

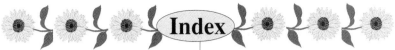
H

Habits, 47, 49, 50, 72
Hair, 13, 18, 125
Happy dispositions, 2
Harmful Foods list, 121
Headaches, 6, 74
Healing crisis, 26
Healing Therapies, 157-160
Herbs, 31, 117, 162
Hearing, 6
Heart, 9-10, 13, 71, 119
  Healthy Heart Habits for, 138
Heartburn, 27
Heimlich Maneuver, 82, 128-131
Herb Teas, 80, 116
High vibration living, 1-4
Homeopathy Therapy, 158
Hyperventilation, 79

I

Immune, 19, 26, 62, 176
Indigestion, 6, 27, 43
Intelligence, 14
Ionization process, 7

J

Joints, 6, 13, 48, 73
Juices, 116-118

K

Kelp, 111
Kidneys, 9, 10, 13, 69

L

Laxatives, 6, 12, 43
Legs, 50-51, 75
Lemon juice, 111
Ligaments, 48

Liquid Aminos, 101, 107, 111
Liver, 9, 13, 43, 70
Longevity, 65, 72, 102, 123, 138, 175, 178
Lungs, 1-4, 7-20, 23, 41-44, 47, 54-58, 60, 64-70, 72-74, 81-83, 98, 101, 107, 133-134, 148, 167, 177

M

Magnesium, 78, 80, 110, 113, 138, 156
Massage, 43, 148, 157-161
Meat, 39, 107-113, 111, 121
Meditation, 13, 84, 135
Memory loss, 6
Menopause, 156
Metabolism, 9, 133
Milk products, 32, 78, 82
Minerals, 78, 111-113, 115, 156
Mold, 17
Mucus, 12, 18, 24-31
Muscles, 13, 25, 47-48, 57
Muscular aches, 6

N

Nasal Sniff Wash & Spray, 78
Natural foods, 24, 91, 119
Naturopathy, 158
Natural Living, 2
Neck, 31
Nerves & system, 9, 13, 44, 77
Nicotine, 19, 23
Nitrates, 77, 123
Nose, 12, 29-31, 66
Nose breathing, 45
Nutrients, 7, 11, 43, 73
Nutrition, 2, 81, 97, 105-106, 114, 116, 119, 121, 152, 157, 159, 161-162, 175

We shall never know all the good that a simple smile can do.

Dream big, think big, but enjoy the small miracles of everyday life.

Index

O

Oils, health, 119, 152, 159
Organic foods, 27, 101, 107-108
Organic minerals, 111, 156
Osteopathy, 158
Osteoporosis, 110, 156
Overweight, 37, 105, 120
Oxygen, 2-20, 23, 27, 29,
    41-45, 47, 53-56, 60, 63-64,
    66, 68, 70-71, 74-75, 77,
    81, 83-84, 91, 95, 98, 101,
    114-115, 124-126, 129,
    133-134, 136-137, 147, 163

P

Pain, 6, 12, 51, 73-74
Painkillers, 6, 12
Pancreas, 43
Peace, 13, 143, 165
Pep drinks, 105, 116
Peristalsis, 43, 146
Pesticides, 18, 108
Phosphorus, 110, 113
Physical, 9, 27, 34, 62, 101, 137
Phytochemicals, 100, 122
Pituitary (master) gland, 44,
    64, 68
Plants, 14, 154
Pneumogastric nerve, 28
Pollens, 17-18, 66
Pollutants, 14, 30, 39, 162
Popcorn Recipe, 116
Pores, 14, 16, 65, 66
Positive thinking, 13
Posture, 46-58, 77, 83, 157,
    159, 175
Pregnancy, 84

Preservatives, 109-111, 121
Product Summary, food, 91
Protein, 102-103, 107, 109,
    113-114, 162

R

Radon, 36-38
Recipes, 106, 116, 118
Reflexes, 56, 158
Reflexology Therapy, 158
Reiki Therapy, 159
Relaxation, 104, 140-142
Respiratory ailments, 6, 12,
    78-79
Rest, 139-142
Rhinitis medicamentosus, 78
Rib cage, 87-88
Rice Casserole Recipe, 106
Rolfing Therapy, 159

S

Salad, 102, 106-107
Salad dressing, 106
Salt, 110 -112
Second Wind, 4
Shiatsu Therapy, 163
Shoulders, 47, 51
Singers, 54
Sinuses, 6, 12, 30-32
Skin, 13, 65, 136, 158
    or third lung, 65-66
Skin tone, 55, 145
Sleep, 45, 79-80, 89, 101,
    105, 136, 139-141
Smog, 91-95
Smoking, 19-24

Eat to live, and not live to eat. Many dishes, many diseases, – Ben Franklin

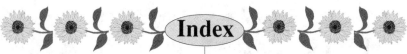

Snacks, 102
Snoring, 32, 81, 162
Sodium nitrate, 109-110, 121
Solar energy, 123, 153-155
Solar Plexus, 44
Spine, Spinal Column, 17, 48-52, 163
Spiritual development, 13-14
Spleen, 43
Sports Therapy, 160
Stomach Exercise, 59
Stress, 2, 13, 38, 45, 89-90, 114
Stretching, 4, 58, 90
Stroke, 22, 97, 145, 147
Sugar, 19, 39, 110, 113, 121
Sulphur Dioxide, 110, 121
Sunshine, 2, 153-155
Supplements, 31, 80, 95, 156
Sweat glands, 12
Swedish Therapy, 160
Swimmers, 53, 97

T

Teeth, 6, 112, 126
Tendons, 13
Thoracic cavity, 16, 17, 41, 43
Throat, 6, 10, 12
Tonsils, 18
Toxic foods, 109-110, 121
Toxic poisons, 7, 10-12, 26, 43, 73-74

Trachea, 15-16
Tragering Therapy, 159
Trichinosis, 109

U

Uric acid, 108
Urine, 10, 113

V

Vegetable Protein Chart, 103
Vegetables, 33, 96, 99, 101-103
Vegetarians, 108-109
Veins Varicose, 8, 10-11, 51, 75
Vinegar, See Apple Cider Vinegar
Vital Nerve Force, 134, 140, 148
Vitamin B-Complex, 78
Vitamin C, 19, 31, 40, 82, 95
Vitamin D, 152
Vitamin E, 96-99, 101, 119, 138

W

Waistline, 16, 49-50
Walking, 47, 50, 75-77, 105, 136, 146
Water, 112, 115-116
Water Therapy, 163
Wheat Germ, 98-99

Y

Yoga, 44-45, 62, 160

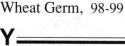

HAVE AN APPLE HEALTHY LIFE!

Man is composed of such elements as vital breath, deeds, thoughts and the senses. – The Upanishads

Perhaps the most valuable result of all education is the ability to make yourself do the thing you have to do, when it ought to be done, as it ought to be done, whether you like it or not!

Where there is great love there are always miracles. – Willa Cather

When you live The Bragg Healthy Lifestyle you can help activate your own powerful internal defense arsenal and maintain it at top efficiency. But, bad or sloppy breathing habits make it harder for your body to fight off illness.

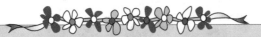

More Praises for This Book and The Bragg Healthy Lifestyle

Rock and roll health is better than rock and roll wealth. Thanks to Bragg, the road ain't a drag. We thank the Braggs for the super smooth going and success on our recent whirlwind 20 city tour of England. – David Polemeni, Boy's Town Band, NJ

I've known the wonderful Bragg Books for over 25 years, when I met Patricia in Hawaii. They are a blessing to me and my family and to all who read them to help make this a healthier world. – Pastor Mike MacIntosh, Horizon Christian Fellowship

After finding the Bragg Vinegar Book in a health food store, I Started making your apple cider vinegar drink 3 times a day, miracles happened – my chronic fatigue is gone! I also suffered from fibromylgia, and had to quit work because of all the pain. Now I can go to work again; after 16 long years of suffering and thousands of dollars I spent trying to get well, I have my life back again. I can never thank you enough! – Fran Covert, Aurora, Colorado

When I was younger (working around asbestos) I inhaled asbestos fibers of which the doctors told me there is no way to clear it up and no cure. I was not feeling well and my chest hurt. A friend I play golf with here in Santa Barbara, CA., introduced me to your Bragg Organic Apple Cider Vinegar Cocktail. I drink it 3 times a day and also use it over my salads. I am now feeling very healthy and strong! What a blessing. I feel 100% better; It's helping me clean out my asbestos fibers. Thanks to my friend, and to you for such a great product and your vinegar book on all the ways to use your healthy vinegar. I will continue to follow your teachings and use your products. – Al Escalera, Santa Barbara, CA

I read your book on uses for Bragg Organic Apple Cider Vinegar and am now taking it daily. After passing on the book to my mom, she too started using your vinegar and found that the pain in her shoulder that had been waking her up at nights for years has vanished. Thank you. – Catherine Cox, Toronto, Ontario, Canada

I am now following your great book, The Bragg Healthy Lifestyle which I heard of through a friend. This Bragg book is a life-changer and has blessed my health and life. It will make wonderful gifts for my friends. – Delphine, Singapore

172

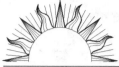

MY DAILY HEALTH JOURNAL

Today is:____/____/____

> **I have said my morning resolve and am ready to practice The Bragg Healthy Lifestyle today and every day.**

Yesterday I went to bed at: Today I arose at: Weight:

Today I practiced the No-Heavy Breakfast or No-Breakfast Plan: ☐ yes ☐ no

- For Breakfast I drank: Time:
  For Breakfast I ate:

      Time:

Supplements:

- For Lunch I ate: Time:

Supplements:

- For Dinner I ate: Time:

Supplements:

- Glasses of Water I Drank during Day:
- List Snacks – Kind and When:

- **I took part in these physical activities today:**

Grade each on scale of 1 to 10 (desired optimum health is 10).
- **I rate my day for the following categories:**

Previous Night's Sleep:	Stress/Anxiety:
Energy Level:	Elimination:
Physical Activity:	Health:
Peacefulness:	Accomplishments:
Happiness:	Self-Esteem:

- **General Comments and To Do List:**

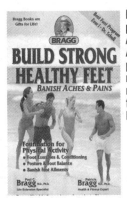
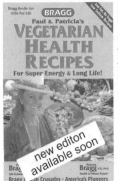
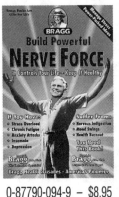
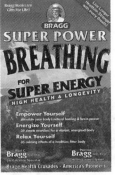

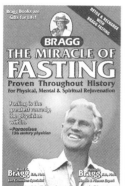
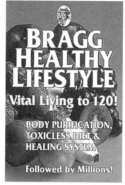
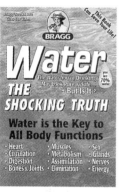
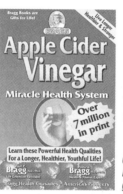
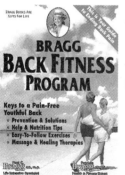
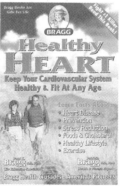

Bragg Organic Raw Apple Cider Vinegar
With the Mother . . . Nature's Delicious, Healthy Miracle

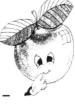
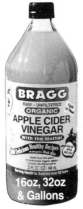

HAVE AN APPLE HEALTHY LIFE!

– IF ? –

Your Favorite Health Store doesn't carry Bragg Products & Books - Ask them to Contact their Distributor to stock them!

Or they can Call Bragg at
1-800-446-1990

BRAGG
RAW – UNFILTERED
ORGANIC
APPLE CIDER VINEGAR
With the Mother

16oz, 32oz & Gallons

INTERNAL BENEFITS:
- Helps Normalize & Control Weight
- Rich in Miracle Potassium & Enzymes
- Natural Antibiotic & Germ Fighter
- Helps Eliminate Toxins & Body Sludge
- Improves Digestion & Balances pH
- Relieves Sore & Dry Throats
- Helps Remove Artery Plaque
- Helps Fight Arthritis & Stiffness

EXTERNAL BENEFITS:
- Helps Promote Youthful, Healthy Body
- Helps Promote & Maintain Healthy Skin
- Soothes Sunburn, Bites & Rashes
- Helps Relieve Dandruff & Itching Scalp
- Helps Heal Acne, Pimples & Shingles
- Soothes Aching Joints & Muscles

BRAGG ALL NATURAL LIQUID AMINOS
Healthy Seasoning Alternative to Tamari & Soy Sauce With 16 Amino Acids

BRAGG LIQUID AMINOS – Nutrition you need...taste you will love...a family favorite for over 88 years. A delicious source of nutritious life-renewing protein from healthy non-GMO soybeans only. Add to or spray over casseroles, tofu, soups, sauces, gravies, potatoes, popcorn, and vegetables, etc. An ideal "pick-me-up" broth at work, home or gym. Health replacement for Tamari, Worchestershire and Soy Sauce. Start today and add 16 vital Amino Acids to your daily diet for healthy living – the easy BRAGG LIQUID AMINOS Way!

SPRAY or DASH brings NEW TASTE DELIGHTS! PROVEN & ENJOYED BY MILLIONS.

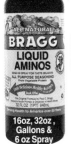

BRAGG LIQUID AMINOS

16oz, 32oz , Gallons & 6 oz Spray

America's Healthiest All-Purpose Seasoning

Certified Non-GMO Soybeans

Spray or Dash of Bragg Aminos Brings New Taste Delights to Season:			Pure Soybeans and Purified Water Only:
• Tempeh	• Dressings	• Soups	■ No Added Sodium
• Tofu	• Gravies	• Rice/Beans	■ No Coloring Agents
• Stir-frys	• Sauces	• Wok foods	■ No Preservatives
• Salads	• Poultry	• Meats	■ Not Fermented
• Veggies	• Fish	• Popcorn	■ No Chemicals
• Casseroles & Potatoes		• Macrobiotics	■ No Additives
			■ No Wheat

BRAGG ORGANIC OLIVE OIL
Delicious, Extra Virgin, Unrefined, First Cold-Pressed

BRAGG ORGANIC OLIVE OIL – is made from 100% organically grown Arbequina Olives that continually provides the best quality and flavor. A heart healthy oil that's an antioxidant oleic acid and vitamin E rich that helps to normalize cholesterol and blood pressure. It has a delicious, smooth body with a light after taste, adding the finest flavor and aroma to salads, vegetables, pastas, pestos, sauces, sautés, potatoes and most foods – even popcorn. Also it's a great skin tonic. In 400 B.C. Hippocrates, the Father of Medicine used and wrote about olive oil's great health benefits.

BRAGG ORGANIC Extra Virgin OLIVE OIL Cold Pressed

16oz, 32oz & Gallons

– Other Bragg Healthy Products for your taste delights:

★ Bragg Sprinkle (herbs & spices)
★ Bragg Organic Kelp Seasoning
★ Bragg Aminos Marinade & Sauce
★ Bragg Salad Dressings:
  ★ Vinaigrette ★ Ginger/Sesame

BRAGG OLIVE OIL VINAIGRETTE OR MARINADE
⅓ cup Bragg Organic Extra Virgin Olive Oil
½ cup Bragg Organic Apple Cider Vinegar
1 tsp Bragg Liquid Aminos (All-Purpose) Seasoning
1 to 2 tsps raw Honey • 1 to 2 cloves Garlic, mince
½ tsp fresh Ginger, grate • ¼ tsp Bragg Sprinkle (herbs & spices)

– Make copies when needed for mailing in. –

Send for Free Health Bulletins

Patricia Bragg wants to keep in touch with you, your relatives and friends about the latest Health, Nutrition, Exercise and Longevity Discoveries. Please enclose one stamp for each USA name listed. Foreign listings send postal reply coupons.

With Blessings of Health, Peace and Thanks,

Patricia

Please make copy, then print clearly and mail to:

BRAGG HEALTH CRUSADES, Box 7, Santa Barbara, CA 93102

You can help too!

Keep the Bragg Health Crusades "Crusading" with your tax-deductible gifts.

Name

Address ______ Apt. No.

City ______ State ______ Zip

Phone ( ) ______ E-mail

Name

Address ______ Apt. No.

City ______ State ______ Zip

Phone ( ) ______ E-mail

Name

Address ______ Apt. No.

City ______ State ______ Zip

Phone ( ) ______ E-mail

Name

Address ______ Apt. No.

City ______ State ______ Zip

Phone ( ) ______ E-mail

Name

Address ______ Apt. No.

City ______ State ______ Zip

Phone ( ) ______ E-mail

Bragg Health Crusades spreading health worldwide since 1912

BRAGG ORGANIC APPLE CIDER VINEGAR

SIZE	PRICE	UPS SHIPPING & HANDLING For USA	$ Amount
16 oz.	$ 2.39 each	S/H – Please add $6 for 1st bottle and $1.50 each additional bottle	•
16 oz.	$23.00 Special Case /12	S/H Cost by Time Zone: CA $8. PST/MST $11. CST $15. EST $17.	•
32 oz.	$ 3.89 each	S/H – Please add $6 for 1st bottle and $2.00 each additional bottle	•
32 oz.	$41.00 Special Case /12	S/H Cost by Time Zone: CA $13. PST/MST $17. CST $24. EST $28.	•
1 gal.	$12.98 each	S/H 1st Bottle: CA $6. PST/MST $8. CST $9. EST $10. + $6 ea add. bottle	•
1 gal.	$47.00 Special Case /4	S/H Cost by Time Zone: CA $12. PST/MST $16. CST $23. EST $27.	•

Bragg Vinegar is a food and not taxable

	$	
Bragg VINEGAR	$	•
Shipping & Handling		•
TOTAL	$	•

BRAGG LIQUID AMINOS

SIZE	PRICE	UPS SHIPPING & HANDLING For USA	$ Amount
6 oz.	$ 2.98 each	S/H – Please add $4.00 for 1st 3 bottles – $1.25 each additional bottle	•
6 oz.	$ 65.00 Special Case /24	S/H Cost by Time Zone: CA $8. PST/MST $9. CST $11. EST $13.	•
16 oz.	$ 3.95 each	S/H – Please add $6 for 1st bottle – $1.25 each additional bottle	•
16 oz.	$ 42.00 Special Case /12	S/H Cost by Time Zone: CA $8. PST/MST $9. CST $13. EST $14.	•
32 oz.	$ 6.45 each	S/H – Please add $6 for 1st bottle – $2.00 each additional bottle	•
32 oz.	$ 70.00 Special Case /12	S/H Cost by Time Zone: CA $11. PST/MST $14. CST $21. EST $27.	•
1 gal.	$ 23.50 each	S/H 1st Bottle: CA $6. PST/MST $8. CST $9. EST $10. + $6 ea add. bottle	•
1 gal.	$ 79.00 Special Case /4	S/H Cost by Time Zone: CA $14. PST/MST $20. CST $25. EST $30.	•

Bragg Aminos is a food and not taxable

	$	
Bragg AMINOS	$	•
Shipping & Handling		•
TOTAL	$	•

BRAGG ORGANIC OLIVE OIL

SIZE	PRICE	USA SHIPPING & HANDLING	$ Amount
16 oz.	$ 8.95 each	S/H – Please add $6 for 1st bottle and $1.50 each additional bottle.	•
16 oz.	$ 95.00 Special Case /12	S/H Cost by Time Zone: CA $8. PST/MST $11. CST $15. EST $17.	•
32 oz.	$ 14.95 each	S/H – Please add $6 for 1st bottle and $2.00 each additional bottle	•
32 oz.	$149.50 Special Case /12	S/H Cost by Time Zone: CA $13. PST/MST $17. CST $24. EST $28.	•
1 gal.	$ 49.95 each	S/H Cost by Time Zone: CA $6. PST/MST $8. CST $9 EST $10.+ $6 ea add. Btl.	•
1 gal.	$169.00 Special Case /4	S/H Cost by Time Zone: CA $12. PST/MST $16. CST $23. EST $27.	•

Bragg Olive Oil is a food and not taxable
Foreign orders, please inquire on postage

Please Specify: ☐ Check ☐ Money Order ☐ Cash
Charge To: ☐ Visa ☐ MasterCard ☐ Discover

	$	
Bragg OLIVE OIL	$	•
Shipping & Handling		•
TOTAL	$	•

Credit Card Number: _____

Card Expires: _____ / _____ month / year

Signature: _____

Business office calls (805) 968-1020. We accept MasterCard, Discover & VISA phone orders. Please prepare order using order form. It speeds your call and serves as order record. Hours: 8 to 4 pm Pacific Time, Monday thru Thursday
● Visit our Web: www.bragg.com ● e-mail: bragg @ bragg.com

CREDIT CARD ORDERS
CALL (800) 446-1990 ☎
OR FAX (805) 968-1001

Mail to: **HEALTH SCIENCE, Box 7, Santa Barbara, CA 93102 USA**
Please Print or Type – Be sure to give street & house number to facilitate delivery.

● Name _____
● Address _____ Apt. No. _____
● City _____ State _____ Zip _____
● Phone ( ) _____ ● E-mail _____

Bragg Products are available at most Health Stores Nationwide.

BOF 505

BRAGG "HOW-TO, SELF-HEALTH" BOOKS

Authored by America's First Family of Health
Live Longer – Healthier – Stronger Self-Improvement Library

Qty. **Bragg Book Titles ORDER FORM** Health Science ISBN 0-87790 Price $ Total

_____ **9 Bragg Book Offer** – Get Healthy, Live Longer – (Vegetarian Recipes not Included) **69.00** | .

_____ **Apple Cider Vinegar** – **Miracle Health System** .... 7.95 | .

_____ **Bragg Healthy Lifestyle** – Vital Living to 120............................... 8.95 _____ .

_____ **Miracle of Fasting** – Bragg Bible of Health for physical rejuvenation .... 9.95 | .

_____ **Healthy Heart & Cardiovascular System** – Have fit heart at any age ... 8.95 | .

_____ **Bragg Back Fitness Program for Pain-Free Strong Back**.................... 8.95 | .

_____ **Water – The Shocking Truth** That Can Save Your Life .... 8.95 | .

_____ **Super Power Breathing** for Super Energy and High Health.................. 8.95 | .

_____ **Build Powerful Nerve Force** – reduce fatigue, stress, anger, anxiety ..... 8.95 | .

_____ **Build Strong Healthy Feet** – Dr. Scholl said *"it's the best"* .... 8.95 | .

NEW Bragg's Vegetarian Health Recipes – Delicious & Nutritious   9.95

TOTAL   (will soon be available)
COPIES   Prices subject to change without notice.   **TOTAL BOOKS $**   .

Please Specify: ☐ Check ☐ Money Order ☐ Cash

CA Residents add sales tax   .

Shipping & Handling   .

Charge To:> ☐ Visa ☐ Master Card ☐ Discover

Month Year
|
Card Expires

VISA   MasterCard   DISCOVER

(USA Funds Only)
TOTAL ENCLOSED $.

USA Shipping | Please add $4 first book $1 each additional book

USA retail book orders over $50 add $6 only

Foreign Shipping | Canada & Foreign orders add $5 first book, $1.50 @ additional book

Credit Card Number

Signature

CREDIT CARD ORDERS ONLY
CALL **(800) 446-1990**
OR FAX **(805) 968-1001**

Business office calls (805) 968-1020. We accept MasterCard, Discover or VISA phone orders. Please prepare order using this order form. It will speed your call and serve as your order record. Hours: 8 to 4 pm Pacific Time, Monday thru Thursday.
Visit our Web: www.bragg.com • e-mail: bragg@bragg.com

See & Order Bragg 'Bound' Books, E-Books, & Products on www.bragg.com
Mail to: **HEALTH SCIENCE, Box 7, Santa Barbara, CA 93102 USA**

Name   BOF505

Address   Apt. No.

City   State   Zip
Phone (   )   E-mail

Bragg Books are available most Health & Book Stores – Nationwide

BRAGG SPRINKLE - Herb & Spice Seasoning

SIZE	PRICE	UPS SHIPPING & HANDLING For USA	$ Amount
2.5 oz.	$ 3.99 each	S/H – Please add $4 for 1st 3 bottles and $1.00 each additional bottle	.
2.5 oz.	$ 43.00 Special Case /12	S/H Cost by Time Zone: CA $5. PST/MST $6. CST $7. EST $9.	.

Bragg Sprinkle is a food and not taxable

	$	
Bragg Sprinkle	$	.
Shipping & Handling		.
TOTAL	$	.

BRAGG KELP–FEAST OF THE SEA

SIZE	PRICE	UPS SHIPPING & HANDLING For USA	$ Amount
1.5 oz.	$ 2.75 each	S/H – Please add $4 for 1st 3 bottles and $1.00 each additional bottle	.
1.5 oz.	$ 30.00 Special Case /12	S/H Cost by Time Zone: CA $5. PST/MST $6. CST $7. EST $9.	.

Bragg Kelp & Salad Dressings are food and not taxable

	$	
Bragg Kelp	$	.
Shipping & Handling		.
TOTAL	$	.

BRAGG SALAD DRESSINGS

SIZE	PRICE	USA SHIPPING & HANDLING	$ Amount
★ Bragg GINGER & SESAME Salad Dressing			
12 oz.	$ 3.99 each	S/H – Please add $6 for 1st bottle and $1.25 each additional bottle	.
12 oz.	$ 43.00 Special Case /12	S/H Cost by Time Zone: CA $8. PST/MST $10. CST $14. EST $16.	.
★ Bragg Organic Vinaigrette Salad Dressing			
12 oz.	$ 4.29 each	S/H – Please add $6 for 1st bottle and $1.25 each additional bottle.	.
12 oz.	$ 47.00 Special Case /12	S/H Cost by Time Zone: CA $8. PST/MST $10. CST $14. EST $16.	.

The NEW Bragg Health Products shown on this page are available most Health Stores or wherever you buy Bragg Health Products.

	$	
Bragg Salad Dressing	$	.
Shipping & Handling		.
TOTAL	$	.

BRAGG LIQUID AMINOS MARINADE & SAUCE

SIZE	PRICE	USA SHIPPING & HANDLING	
Bragg Liquid Aminos Marinade & Sauce			.
12 oz.	$ 4.29 each	S/H – Please add $6 for 1st bottle and $1.25 each additional bottle.	
12 oz.	$ 47.00 Special Case /12	S/H Cost by Time Zone: CA $8. PST/MST $10. CST $14. EST $16.	

Bragg Marinade is a food and not taxable

	$	
Bragg Salad Dressing	$	.
Shipping & Handling		.
TOTAL	$	.

Foreign orders, please inquire on postage

Please Specify: ☐ Check ☐ Money Order ☐ Cash
Charge To: ☐ Visa ☐ MasterCard ☐ Discover

Credit Card Number: _____

Card Expires: ___ / ___ month / year

Signature: _____

Business office calls (805) 968-1020. We accept MasterCard, Discover & VISA phone orders. Please prepare order using order form. It speeds your call and serves as order record. Hours: 8 to 4 pm Pacific Time, Monday thru Thursday
• Visit our Web: www.bragg.com • e-mail: bragg @ bragg.com

CREDIT CARD ORDERS
CALL (800) 446-1990 ☎
OR FAX (805) 968-1001

Mail to: **HEALTH SCIENCE, Box 7, Santa Barbara, CA 93102 USA**   BOF 605
Please Print or Type – Be sure to give street & house number to facilitate delivery.

Name _____
Address _____ Apt. No. _____
City _____ State _____ Zip _____
Phone ( ) _____ E-mail _____

Bragg Products are available at most Health Stores.

BRAGG "HOW-TO, SELF-HEALTH" BOOKS

Authored by America's First Family of Health
Live Longer – Healthier – Stronger Self-Improvement Library

Qty.	Bragg Book Titles ORDER FORM Health Science ISBN 0-87790	Price	$ Total
_____	**9 Bragg Book Offer** – Get Healthy, Live Longer – (Vegetarian Recipes not Included)	**69.00**	•
_____	**Apple Cider Vinegar** – **Miracle Health System**	7.95	•
_____	**Bragg Healthy Lifestyle** – Vital Living to 120..	8.95	•
_____	**Miracle of Fasting** – Bragg Bible of Health for physical rejuvenation	9.95	•
_____	**Healthy Heart & Cardiovascular System** – Have fit heart at any age ...	8.95	•
_____	**Bragg Back Fitness Program for Pain-Free Strong Back**....................	8.95	•
_____	**Water** – **The Shocking Truth** That Can Save Your Life	8.95	•
_____	**Super Power Breathing** for Super Energy and High Health..................	8.95	•
_____	**Build Powerful Nerve Force** – reduce fatigue, stress, anger, anxiety	8.95	•
_____	**Build Strong Healthy Feet** – Dr. Scholl said *"it's the best"*	8.95	•

	NEW Bragg's Vegetarian Health Recipes – Delicious & Nutritious	9.95

TOTAL COPIES   (will soon be available)
Prices subject to change without notice.

TOTAL BOOKS $ •

Please Specify: ☐ Check ☐ Money Order ☐ Cash

CA Residents add sales tax	•
Shipping & Handling	•

Charge To: ☐ Visa ☐ Master Card ☐ Discover

(USA Funds Only)
TOTAL ENCLOSED $ •

Month   Year

| VISA | MasterCard | DISCOVER |

Card Expires

USA Shipping	Please add $4 first book $1 each additional book

USA retail book orders over $50 add $6 only

Credit Card Number

Foreign Shipping	Canada & Foreign orders add $5 first book, $1.50 @ additional book

Signature

See & Order Bragg 'Bound' Books, E-Books, & Products on www.bragg.com
Mail to: **HEALTH SCIENCE, Box 7, Santa Barbara, CA 93102 USA**

Name _____   BOF505

Address _____   Apt. No. _____

City _____   State _____   Zip _____

Phone (   )   E-mail

Send for Free Health Bulletins

Patricia Bragg wants to keep in touch with you, your relatives and friends about the latest Health, Nutrition, Exercise and Longevity Discoveries. Please enclose one stamp for each USA name listed. Foreign listings send postal reply coupons.

With Blessings of Health and Thanks,

Patricia

Please make copy, then print clearly and mail to:

BRAGG HEALTH CRUSADES, Box 7, Santa Barbara, CA 93102
You can help too!
Keep the Bragg Health Crusades "Crusading" with your tax-deductible gifts.

Name

Address   Apt. No.

City   State   Zip

Phone (   )   E-mail

Name

Address   Apt. No.

City   State   Zip

Phone (   )   E-mail

Name

Address   Apt. No.

City   State   Zip

Phone (   )   E-mail

Name

Address   Apt. No.

City   State   Zip

Phone (   )   E-mail

Name

Address   Apt. No.

City   State   Zip

Phone (   )   E-mail

Bragg Health Crusades spreading health worldwide since 1912

PATRICIA BRAGG, N.D., Ph.D.
Health Crusader & Angel of Health & Healing

**Author, Lecturer, Nutritionist, Health Educator & Fitness Advisor
to World Leaders, Hollywood Stars, Singers, Dancers, Athletes, etc.**

Patricia is a 100% dedicated health crusader with a passion like her father, Paul C. Bragg, world renowned health authority. Patricia has won international fame on her own in this field. She conducts Health and Fitness Seminars for Conventions and Women's, Men's, Youth and Church Groups around the world and promotes The Bragg Healthy Lifestyle Living and "How-To, Self-Health" Books on Radio Talk Shows throughout the English-speaking world. Consultants to Presidents and Royalty, to Stars of Stage, Screen and TV and to Champion Athletes, Patricia and her father co-authored The Bragg Health Library of Instructive, Inspiring Books that promote a healthier lifestyle, for a long, vital, happy life.

Patricia herself is the symbol of health, perpetual youth and radiant, feminine energy. She is a living and sparkling example of her and her father's healthy lifestyle precepts and this she loves sharing world-wide.

A fifth-generation Californian on her mother's side, Patricia was reared by The Bragg Natural Health Method from infancy. In school, she not only excelled in athletics, but also won honors for her studies and her counseling. She is an accomplished musician and dancer . . . as well as tennis player and mountain climber . . . and the youngest woman ever to be granted a U.S. Patent. Patricia is a popular gifted Health Teacher and a dynamic, in-demand Talk Show Guest where she spreads the simple, easy-to-follow Bragg Healthy Lifestyle for everyone of all ages.

Man's body is his vehicle through life, his earthly temple . . . and the Creator wants us filled with joy & health for a long fruitful life. The Bragg Crusades of Health and Fitness (3 John 2) has carried her around the world over 13 times – spreading physical, spiritual, emotional and mental health and joy. Health is our birthright and Patricia teaches how to prevent the destruction of our health from man-made wrong habits of living.

Patricia's been a Health Consultant to American Presidents and British Royalty, to Betty Cuthbert, Australia's "Golden Girl," who holds 16 world records and four Olympic gold medals in women's track and to New Zealand's Olympic Track and Triathlete Star, Allison Roe. Among those who come to her for advice are some of Hollywood's top Stars from Clint Eastwood to the ever-youthful singing group, The Beach Boys and their families, Singing Stars of the Metropolitan Opera and top Ballet Stars. Patricia's message is of world-wide appeal to people of all ages, nationalities and walks-of-life. Those who follow The Bragg Healthy Lifestyle and attend the Bragg Crusades world-wide are living testimonials . . . like ageless, super athlete, Jack LaLanne, who at age 15 went from sickness to Total Health!